A Practical Guide to Therapeutic Communication for Health Professionals

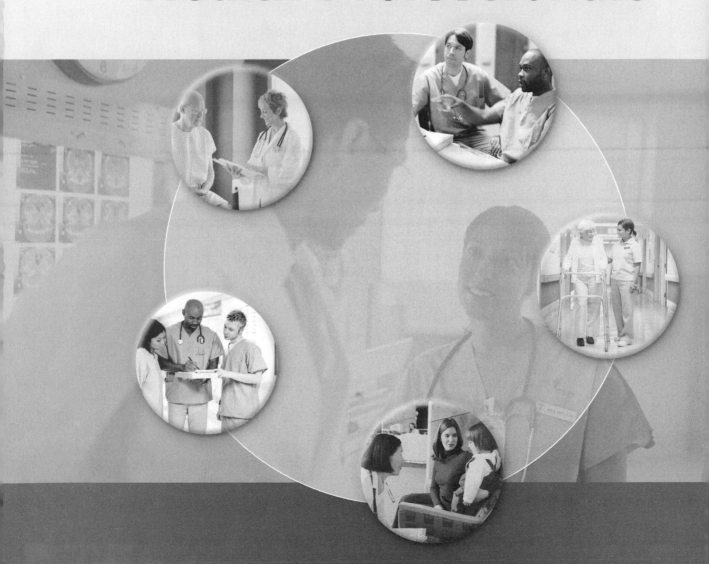

evolve

To access your Instructor Resources, visit:

http://evolve.elsevier.com/Hosley/communications/

Evolve Student Learning Resources for **Julie Hosley and Elizabeth Molle: A Practical Guide to Therapeutic Communication for Health Professionals, ed 1** offers the following features:

Student Resources

- **Communication Surfer Exercises**
  from the text enable students to easily complete these activities online.

- **Weblinks**
  links to websites carefully chosen to supplement the content of the textbook.

A Practical Guide to Therapeutic Communication for Health Professionals

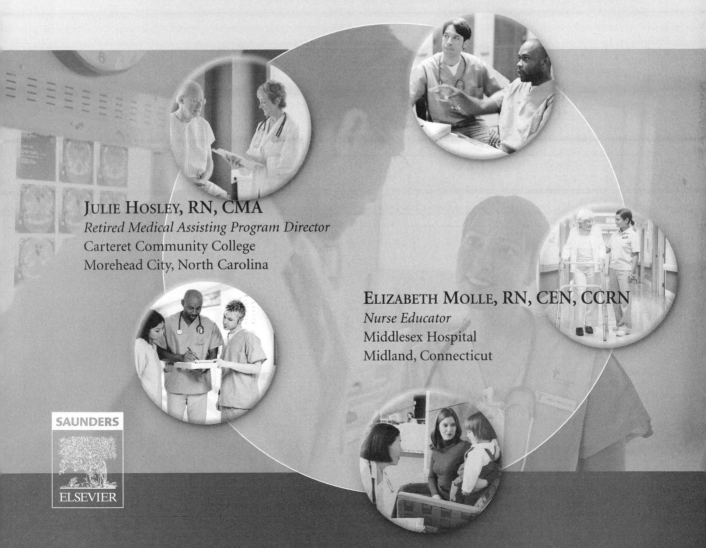

JULIE HOSLEY, RN, CMA
Retired Medical Assisting Program Director
Carteret Community College
Morehead City, North Carolina

ELIZABETH MOLLE, RN, CEN, CCRN
Nurse Educator
Middlesex Hospital
Midland, Connecticut

SAUNDERS

ELSEVIER

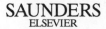

SAUNDERS
ELSEVIER

11830 Westline Industrial Drive
St. Louis, Missouri 63146

A PRACTICAL GUIDE TO THERAPEUTIC COMMUNICATION   ISBN-13: 978-1-4160-0000-6
FOR HEALTH PROFESSIONALS   ISBN-10: 1-4160-0000-3
Copyright © 2006, Elsevier Inc.

ISBN-13: 978-1-4160-0000-6
ISBN-10: 1-4160-0000-3

Acquisitions Editor: Michael S. Ledbetter
Developmental Editor: Celeste Clingan
Publishing Services Manager: Melissa Lastarria
Project Manager: Andrea Campbell
Design Project Manager: Bill Drone

Working together to grow
libraries in developing countries

www.elsevier.com | www.bookaid.org | www.sabre.org

ELSEVIER   BOOK AID International   Sabre Foundation

Printed in the United States of America
Last digit is the print number: 9 8 7 6 5

Thanks to my family for always believing in me.

Julie Hosley

I would like to dedicate this book to my dear friend Julie. You are a great co-author and friend. We have been through a lot in these past years. I admire your strength and courage. I wish you the very best. Enjoy your retirement!

Elizabeth Molle

PREFACE

Welcome to *A Practical Guide to Therapeutic Communication for Health Professionals*. We hope this text will make it easier for you to interact and communicate in the medical field. We have drawn from our combined over-sixty years of communication experiences to give you the tools needed to become a successful health care professional.

We designed this text to approach communication in an easily understandable and interesting format. Communication is a learned skill. This book will help you to improve your communication skills with your patients and coworkers. You will read about various communication theories and challenges followed by suggestions and guidelines to help you work your way to effective communication. Not all of the suggestions will work or are necessary in all situations, but the majority of the items have helped us through many rewarding years as health care professionals. We hope they will be helpful to you as well.

We filled the text with features that we hope will make the topic of communication as interesting to you as it is to us. These include:

- *Learning objectives* to alert you to the skills or knowledge you should gain from each chapter.
- *Key terms* to introduce you to words or concepts that may not be familiar to you.
- *Communication IQ* review to highlight areas of communication in which you might be weak.
- *Idiom cartoons* to show you how commonly used phrases may interfere with effective communication.
- *Legal Eagle* to reinforce to you that medical information is private and confidential with both ethical and legal implications.
- *Spotlight on Success* to remind you that the foundations you establish as a student will help you build a rewarding career.
- *Taking the Chapter to Work* to give you examples of compassionate, caring health care professionals working through everyday interactions.
- *Assignment Board* to help you keep track of assignments with a handy check-off list.
- *Checking Your Comprehension* to direct you back through the chapter to points you may need to reinforce.
- *Critical Thinking exercises* to expand your mind with probing questions that have no clear-cut, black or white answers.
- *Communication Surfer exercises* to introduce you to the ever-growing information available to you and your patients through Internet technology.

As you work your way through this text, keep in mind that the skills you gain now will make health care a rewarding career for many years to come.

CONTENTS

1

INTRODUCTION TO COMMUNICATION: BUILDING THE FRAMEWORK

LEARNING OBJECTIVES

Upon successful completion of this chapter, you will be able to:

- Describe the steps in effective communication.
- List your responsibilities in the communication process.
- List the patient's responsibilities in the communication process.
- Differentiate between verbal and nonverbal communication.
- Explain how nonverbal communication can affect the interpretation of verbal messages.
- Describe ways to determine when touch is welcome or appropriate.
- List ways to establish and maintain rapport with patients.
- Explain how sympathy and empathy differ.

KEY TERMS

Clarify, Clarification, Clarifying	HIPAA	Preparatory
Colloquialisms	Incongruent, Incongruence	Proxemics
Compliant, Compliance, Complying	Idiom	Rapport
Credible	Kinesics	Spatial
Dynamics	Maintenance	Sympathy
Empathy	Massage	Validate, Validation, Validating
Feedback	Orient, Orientation	Verify, Verification, Verifying
	Paralanguage	

Test Your Communication IQ

Before reading this chapter, complete this short self-assessment test. Decide which statements are true and which are false.

1. The health care worker should maintain control of the conversation to keep communication brief and to the point.
2. Using the patient's first name makes him more comfortable and promotes rapport.
3. Nonverbal communication is often as important as verbal communication.
4. Effective communication is the key to good patient care.
5. Saying, "You'll be just fine," is reassuring to patients and is a good therapeutic response.
6. Using proper medical terminology will impress your patients and should be used whenever possible.
7. Tapping your patient on the shoulder for good luck is an appropriate use of touch.

Results

Statements three and four are true; all others are false. How did you do? Read the chapter to find more information on these topics.

INTRODUCTION TO COMMUNICATION: BUILDING THE FRAMEWORK

Communication is vital to our survival. It fills the practical need of transmitting our wants and needs to those who can fill them for us and helps us respond to the wants and needs of others. Good communication also helps meet our social needs; it gives us pleasure and relief from stress and forms bonds with others in our group to increase our sense of belonging. Communication is easier for some people than for others, but with practice, everyone can learn the steps to better communication. Because we typically spend more than half of our waking hours communicating with others, this skill should be practiced and refined to be more effective, pleasurable, and rewarding.

The ability to communicate and interact effectively is a critical skill for all allied health professionals because of the many barriers and challenges unique to the profession. In this text, we describe ways to serve your patients and your health care career through therapeutic communication. We will help you to understand and be understood in the many areas of health care and in the difficult and puzzling situations that you will confront during your career. Many of the tips and suggestions are helpful for purely social conversations and interactions, but you will find that communicating with persons who are ill, or who are stressed by caring for those who are ill, requires skills far more advanced than those we use in everyday social interaction. Even patients visiting the physician for nothing more than a routine physical examination frequently need help communicating in a stressful and potentially difficult situation. Patients usually spend more relaxed time with you than with the physician, and in most instances they see you as more approachable and more open to communication.

Box **1-1**   **Confidentiality, HIPAA, and You**

The importance of patient confidentiality has been an issue in health care since the earliest concept of one person caring for another. The 2000-year-old Hippocratic Oath (or Oath of Hippocrates), a part of the graduation ceremony for physicians, emphasizes the importance of guarding patient information with the following statement:

"All that may come to my knowledge in the exercise of my profession or outside of my profession or in daily commerce with men, which ought not to be spread abroad, I will keep secret and will never reveal."

The patient's right to privacy is so important that it is included in every specialty's code of ethics. However, until recently, a breach of confidentiality was not punishable by law unless it resulted in damage to a person's reputation, which is called *defamation of character*. This covers both slander (the spoken word) and libel (putting damaging information into print). Other forms of confidentiality breaches that were less damaging were considered lapses in good judgment and were unethical, but no penalties were imposed.

A Congressional effort to help patients maintain health coverage when jobs changed or ended resulted in the Health Insurance Portability and Accountability Act of 1996, or **HIPAA**. It was developed to improve the quality of health care, to keep down spiraling costs, and to protect patients from disclosure of medical information without written, informed consent. The problem of guarding confidentiality in systems with multiple points of access was becoming critical with electronic transmission of sensitive patient information. Insurance companies, health maintenance organizations (HMOs), and other interested parties had access to health information that most of us would prefer not to share.

HIPAA applies to any health information created and maintained in any health care agency or body that compiles and maintains patient information. The Department of Health and Human Services (DHHS) issued a regulation called "The Standard for Privacy of Individually Identifiable Health Information" and established the Office of Civil Rights (OCR) to implement and enforce compliance with the HIPAA guidelines.

At the adoption of the HIPAA, any successfully prosecuted breach of confidentiality is punishable by a variety of fines, ranging from $100 for each violation to $250,000 for selling or using information for improper purposes [Sections 1176(a)(1) and 1177(b)(3) of Public Law 104-191]. Imprisonment ranges up to 10 years for the maximum penalty.

Clearly, keeping your patient's health care information confidential is no longer just an ethical issue; it is now a matter of law.

The information you receive while talking with patients must be transmitted accurately, appropriately, and confidentially (Box 1-1) to physicians and other professional staff members. You must also translate information from physicians and other staff members in a manner that patients can understand. A positive attitude, pleasant presentation, and good communication skills establish **rapport**, a relationship of trust and understanding, for future interactions with patients. These skills also help maintain the flow of communication back and forth between health care professionals.

HOW COMMUNICATION WORKS

Communication at any level forms a bond or connection with another person or persons for an exchange that should benefit at least one of the participants. Ideally, all participants should be equally involved in the message for the best outcome. If one of the participants is not interested in the information, or does not place a value on it, the process of communication may not be complete. For example, think about times you needed to talk to a friend about a problem you hoped she would understand. If she was distracted or did not care to listen, you probably were understandably hurt and frustrated and may not try to confide in her again. Patients feel the same way if they suspect we do not value their concerns.

To be effective, we must determine the information to transmit, choose the best way to send the message, and receive and interpret the responses in the exchange. All forms of communication require the following elements:

• A message to be transmitted in a form understandable to the receiver
• A sender, usually a person, to transmit the message
• A method for transmitting the message—verbal, nonverbal, or written
• A ready and receptive receiver to accept the message
• **Clarification** or **verification** that the message was received and understood

The message will not work in a form the receiver cannot understand. If you transmit a message in English to someone who speaks only another language, if you speak above the patient's comprehension level, or if she cannot or will not hear you, none of the communication elements will work. If the message is not clear or well defined, the exchange is more difficult. For example, how can the patient respond when your message contains very little that he understands, or how will you respond when the physician gives you instructions that make no sense to you? In these cases, the message was not transmitted in an understandable form and communication is incomplete.

The channel or method of transmitting the message may be either spoken or written, it may be body language, or it may be a simple facial expression. We have all transmitted messages to someone across a room using only significant looks and body language. For the message to be transmitted effectively, the receiver must be ready and able to accept it. This is like sending a fax if the receiving machine is not on. If the patient is not ready to accept the message, or cannot receive it because of her physical or emotional state, her "receiver" is not on. In Chapter 2, "Challenges to Communication," we cover how to determine when the patient is "ready to receive" and how to communicate if he is not ready but you need to talk with him about his health care at the time.

When a message has been transmitted, we should be able to determine whether it was received by clarification or verification responses. Recognizing these responses may be as simple as interpreting the receiver's body language, facial expression, or a head nod that the message was received. We may simply see it in the patient's eyes. The verification response may also be as complex as a lengthy and involved written or verbal response.

When the message is in the verbal or spoken form, the sender and receiver alternate roles as they transmit their part of the information needed in the exchange and look for responses in the form of feedback and verification. The process of message exchange is like a tennis match, with the message, like a ball, passing from person to person. Figure 1-1 illustrates the flow of oral communication and its common components.

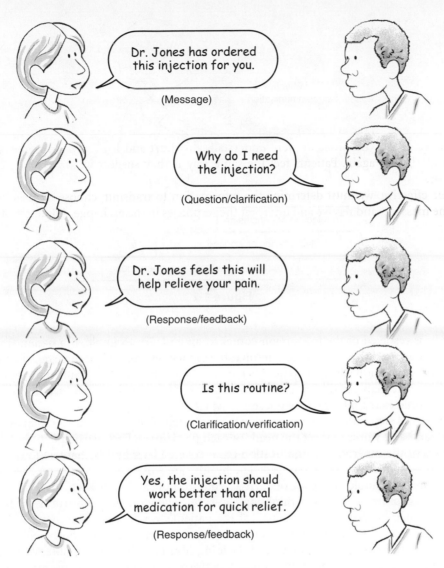

Figure 1-1

Steps in the Communication Process

Communication is conducted in steps (Fig. 1-2). The first is the **preparatory**, introductory, or **orientation** step. This step introduces the participants to each other and helps form a mutual agreement to exchange information. Roles and responsibilities are established within the first few moments, usually by implied agreement. There is usually no formal agreement that each participant will perform certain functions in the exchange, but by founding the relationship, each participant agrees to fulfill his or her part of the exchange until the

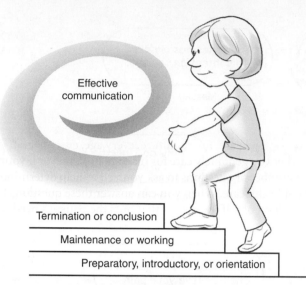

Figure 1-2

situation is resolved or the interaction comes to an end. For example, if a patient makes a health care request that you can help resolve, the guidelines are implied that she will give you all of the information you need to help her. By coming to her aid, you imply that you will do everything reasonable to fill her needs. The two of you have reached an informal agreement, which completes the introductory phase.

The second step is the working, or **maintenance,** step. The conversation is focused on the task at hand and works to meet the needs of each participant. Each participant observes the responses of the other for communication cues (covered later in this chapter) to determine that all messages are properly received. The health care worker usually *directs*, or leads, the interaction but should not control it. It is your responsibility to keep the exchange on track—to keep the patient from rambling—but *controlling* the flow interrupts the free and open exchange needed to determine all of the patient's needs. Today, he may need to talk about his personal problems rather than participate in an intense and comprehensive health history, and you must respect that need. Helping him talk about his problems may be as therapeutic as any clinical procedure you may perform, but gentle, tactful, probing questions (covered in Chapter 3, "Gathering Information") may help guide him back on track to direct the conversation toward his immediate health care needs.

The final step is the termination or conclusion. If the exchange was effective and success-ful, each party is satisfied that messages were transmitted and received as intended. (Guidelines to help overcome a breakdown in communication are covered in Chapter 2, "Challenges to Communication"). At the conclusion of the exchange, goals should be reached, such as determining the patient's current need for care, or, if you are working in an intermediate position, the relationship is transferred to another worker. The relationship may be as short-term as greeting patients for a one-time visit, or may be an established rela-tionship for long-term, chronic care. In either case, or in any health care situation, the **dynamics** of communication—how communication works—and the need for exchange remain the same. All of the steps listed above are involved in any exchange, from a brief conversation as you greet your patients to a complicated transfer of complex medical information over an extended period. If the relationship is long-term, well-established, and pleasant for both the patient and you, at its eventual end you may feel a sense of loss, but you should also feel pride in the independence and growth you have helped your patient achieve.

Your Responsibility to the Patient

Before you can communicate effectively with anyone else, you must first communicate with yourself and understand who you are. Every culture, every age, every person you come in contact with will sense whether you genuinely care for his or her welfare, or if your interest is insincere. Box 1-2 outlines a number of questions to ask yourself to help determine whether you are ready for the demands of health care. When you can answer these questions honestly and selflessly, you have reached a level of self-awareness that puts the patient's needs before your own.

As you interview or interact with patients, you are responsible for keeping conversations focused on the topics at hand. Patients should be allowed to talk about any concerns related to their health, but if they begin to ramble from the subject, you should gently move them back to the main concern. Your other responsibilities for ensuring good communication include the following points:

- Be familiar with the patient's history and current condition to determine what information is needed with the background already available. You need answers to questions such as: Is this simply an annual examination, or is the visit in response to a life-threatening situation? How ill is the patient now? Is he too sick for effective communication?
- Check the patient's history for possible barriers to communication, such as English as a second language, hearing impairment, and so on. Do you need an interpreter? Do you need a notepad for a written exchange?

Box **1-2**   **Are You Ready?**

To determine whether you are ready for the demands of health care, ask yourself these questions:
- Do you genuinely like who you are?
- Are you convinced you have made the right career choice?
- Do you mind being up close and personal with people of all ages, races, ethnic groups, and socioeconomic levels?
- Can you accept differences in cultures, religions, races, and morals and see these as interesting alternatives, not as threatening or inferior?
- Are you distant and detached, or do you give too much and have nothing left for yourself?
- Can you be firm but gentle when you need to be?
- Can you help your patient find his inner strength and then let go?
- Can you keep your personal life and concerns to yourself?
- If the relationship and rapport break down, can you work to resolve the problem, and then recognize and apologize for your part in it?
- When you find yourself disliking a person, can you determine why and rise above it?
- Do you resent taking orders or submitting to authority?

- Be aware of the patient's communication needs. Use common sense and good judgment. Does she need to talk today to relieve stress and anxiety, or is a casual conversation enough for today? Is superficial chatter a cover for more important information? If so, can you determine what she is trying not to tell you?
- Demonstrate courtesy and compassion. Even a brief encounter requires good manners and a caring attitude.
- Remain objective regarding personal and cultural differences. It is not necessary to agree with patients to understand their needs or to provide excellent care. Use your personal differences as a learning opportunity.
- **Clarify** the message for understanding. Did the patient say what you thought he said? Did he understand what you said? Ask or answer as many questions as needed for clarification.
- **Validate** the patient's feelings. She has a right to feel as she does: sad, angry, frightened, and so forth.
- Phrase your message so that patients can understand. Are you using terms above or below the patient's understanding? Are you trying to interact professionally, or are you trying to impress?
- Encourage good health care choices and independent care. It is our goal to turn the patient's care over to him when he is able. Did you use every opportunity to educate him in proper wellness measures?
- Provide **feedback** and ask for it in return to be sure the messages were clearly received. Can the patient repeat your instructions satisfactorily and demonstrate understanding? Did you understand what she was trying to tell you?
- Provide learning tools, such as pamphlets or written instructions for self-care, and be sure they are designed for the patient's needs (see Chapter 4, "Educating Patients").
    See the Legal Eagle box for a discussion of some legal aspects of patient communication.

 ## LEGAL EAGLE

Communication between patients and health care workers must be honest, ethical, and legal. The following points will help keep you within the proper limits:

- Discuss information only within the guidelines set for your scope of practice. You do not have the training and knowledge for in-depth explanations of complex medical information. Many of the patient's concerns must be handled by the physician. Formal protocol and common sense should help you determine what you can and cannot discuss with your patients.
- It is not within your scope of practice to inform patients of their diagnosis or prognosis. If patients ask you these questions, refer them to the physician.
- Patient education must follow the physician's instructions and guidelines and may begin only at the physician's direction.
- Diagnostic testing results (i.e., radiology or laboratory) may not be given to patients without the physician's direct permission.
- Absolutely no patient information can be shared with family members, or with anyone else, without specific patient consent (see Box 1-1, "Confidentiality, HIPAA, and You").

The Patient's Responsibility to You

Patients should be active partners in any communication or exchange. Each participant shares responsibility in keeping lines of communication open and clear of interference and misunderstanding. Our goal is to include patients in as many decisions as possible to help them feel in control of their health. Passive patients, who simply sit and listen, rarely make a conscious effort to restore or maintain health; they rely on their health care providers to do it for them. Active participants feel at least partially in control and are more likely to follow directions. Active participation begins with a truthful and in-depth interview (see Chapter 3, "Gathering Information"). The patient's responsibilities include the following:

- Being truthful and open regarding concerns. We cannot treat patients effectively if they withhold information or do not tell the truth.
- Providing a full medical history regardless of how reluctant they may be to share potentially embarrassing information. Hiding parts of the health history may result in improper treatment. Health care professionals cannot force information that patients refuse to give, but the physician must be informed of areas that need to be discussed further.
- Participating in independent care as much as possible. Most health care should be self-care.
- Complying with health care directions designed to promote wellness. Patients must do their share to maintain health or to ensure a return to an acceptable level of wellness.

There is a strong connection between the quality of a patient's relationship with his health care providers and his **compliance** with prescribed treatment. He must respect those in charge of his care. If he does not feel that you have his best interests at heart, he is less likely to follow prescribed care. He must expect that his information will be held in the strictest confidence and will be used only to design a plan of care for his benefit. Therapeutic communication is the key to this relationship.

HOW WE COMMUNICATE

Using Words: Verbal Communication

Verbal communication exchanges messages using words or language; it is the form we use most often. It includes both oral and written communication. Good verbal communication skills are vital when performing such tasks as instructing, caring for, and educating patients or caregivers, sharing information with the physician or other members of the health care team, and documenting in medical records.

Oral Communication

We send and receive oral, or spoken, communication in health care more often than any other form of communication, making your manner of speaking important in any exchange. The language you use as a professional must be pleasant, polite, and grammatically correct; slang and **colloquialisms** (regional language or terms) may be fun to use in an informal setting but usually are not proper in health care. Chatting with your patient as you establish the early relationship gives you clues that will help you through the interaction. Listen to your patient's grammatical structure, pronunciation, and general manner of speaking to determine her level of education and knowledge, and then use terms she will understand. Patients with higher levels of education will understand and expect correct medical terms;

other patients may be confused by the same phrases. You may find that colloquialisms are a necessary means of communicating with certain patients. By listening carefully to a patient, for example, you should be able to determine her regional or cultural background. Patients from lower socioeconomic classes may be intimidated by medical personnel and find it hard to communicate openly; conversely, highly educated patients may intimidate you and keep you from communicating effectively. Knowing this information helps gauge the appropriate questions, responses, and explanations. For example, you may ask yourself, "Will this patient understand 'cerebrovascular accident' or should I use 'stroke'?" Remember, medical terminology is literally a foreign language, based on Greek and Latin. You would not presume that a Spanish-speaking patient understands English; do not presume that an English-speaking patient understands medical terminology. Are you trying to communicate with the patient or impress him with your education? Phrase your communication appropriately without talking down to the patient.

Other components of the exchange affect the meaning of oral communication. These include non-language sounds and **paralanguage**, or paralinguistics (Box 1-3). These terms are combined in some sources as *nonverbal cues*. Non-language sounds include sighing, humming, chuckling, or laughing. These are sounds in addition to the spoken word. Paralanguage includes quality, volume, pitch, and tone of voice and is applied to the spoken word. Paralanguage and non-language are frequently more important than the verbal exchange. We have less conscious control over paralanguage and non-language. For instance, our voices tend to rise in pitch when we are tense or upset, no matter how hard we try to appear calm. Our voices may tremble when we are sad or angry, or the quality may sound harsh, even if we try to cover our emotions. Our patients will be equally conflicted in words and underlying emotion and can give us clues to concerns they are reluctant to share during the conversation. If nonverbal cues are inconsistent with the message—called **incongruence**—there is a breakdown in communication. The patient may not be filling her part of the mutual agreement to exchange truthful information. You will need to spend more time and effort with this patient to determine what she is trying not to tell you. We cannot help our patients if we treat only the obvious signs and not the underlying concerns that may not be shared.

Written Communication

Written communication obviously uses written language to exchange messages. Since words are used in the exchange, written communication is considered verbal communication

Box **1-3**   **Communicating with Both Sides of the Brain**

Although we use both halves, or hemispheres, of our brain to communicate, the left side of our brain is responsible for language and logic, and the right side processes emotions. We know that the left brain is linked to the right side of the body, and the right brain is linked to the left side. Therefore, the left side, or language/logic side, seems to have better control of the facial expression on the right side of the face. Conversely, our right brain, or emotional side, controls the left side of the face. Theoretically, in an emotional situation, we are less able to control the muscles on the left side of our face. Observing the whole person—posture, gestures, paralanguage, non-language, etc—is very important, but if the message seems incongruent, check the left side of the face for the most uncensored message.

(see Chapter 7, "Writing For Communication"). Clear, concise, accurate communication in any form is important in all areas of health care. This includes exchanges between health care professionals, such as chart notes and memos, as well as communication between patients and professionals. Patients generally receive instructions first as verbal communication, as you or the physician explains points of concern regarding health care. Written instructions then reinforce and remind patients of instructions and explanations. If your patient has poor reading skills or has any barrier to communication, verbal or written, and the instructions are not clear, the meaning may be misinterpreted. This in turn may interfere with treatment and delay recovery. You are responsible for making sure that information was received and understood as it was intended.

Methods for recognizing and overcoming common barriers to communication are covered in Chapter 2, "Challenges to Communication." Educating at the patient's level is covered in Chapter 4, "Educating Patients."

Using Body Language: Nonverbal Communication

Body language—exchanging messages without words—is a form of nonverbal communication. A wide range of behaviors is included in the nonverbal categories of **kinesics** and **proxemics**.

Kinesics

Kinesics involves body movements, such as gestures, posture and body cues, eye movements and facial expressions, and tone and rate of speech. Kinesics reveal inner feelings, such as sadness, happiness, fear, or anger, that may not be apparent in the spoken word. In fact, many emotions are expressed best by nonverbal language. Emotions such as anger, fear, and surprise usually are projected first and best without words, before we have time to hide our emotions. Gestures also have many meanings. Squirming, shrinking away, and fidgeting may mean intense discomfort, perhaps with your line of questioning, if your patient does not appear to be in obvious physical discomfort. Nodding your head, a common gesture, communicates a positive response and lets patients know you are listening. With straight posture, heads up, and eyes forward, patients radiate good health and self-esteem; slumped posture with restricted movements and eyes downcast projects pain, ill-health, or poor self-esteem.

Eyes often hint at what we think and feel. Maintaining friendly eye contact with patients shows interest, warmth, and concern. As you observe your patients during the communication process, watch closely for messages you read in their eyes. "Eye messages" are hardest to hide and may be the easiest to read. Patients who do not maintain eye contact may be impatient, may lack interest in the topic, or may be overwhelmed by information. However, patients from cultures other than North America may feel that maintaining eye contact is rude, challenging, or even sexually suggestive. Eye contact maintained for too long is inappropriate and disturbing and may be interpreted as staring. Be careful as you maintain eye contact if your patient seems uncomfortable.

Since some patients try to mask their feelings, nonverbal communication may carry more meaning than verbal communication. Learn to read what is concealed, as well as what is spoken. Remember that facial expressions (Fig. 1-3) are so important in medicine that tribal doctors used elaborately carved facial masks in their healing rituals for more years than current traditional medicine has existed.

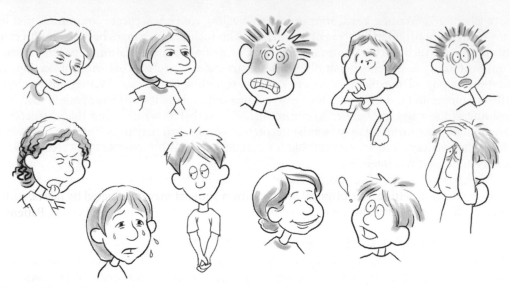

Figure 1-3
Many feelings are obvious to the observant health care worker.

Patients also are very aware of your facial and nonverbal reactions to what they say. Watch your body language to resist transmitting closure (i.e., arms crossed over your chest), distance (i.e., leaning away from the patient or turning your back), or rejection (i.e., frowning, looking away). Facial expressions also may cue patients to the response that you expect or would prefer to hear, such as a report that the treatment is working, whether or not this is true. For example, you ask Mrs. Smith if the latest prescription is working and she responds that she does not think it is. If you look surprised, she may change her answer to please you. Many patients try to anticipate what they think you want to hear and will alter their responses to satisfy you. If you register shock or rejection, you may immediately close all channels of communication between you and the patient, and it may be difficult to reestablish a working relationship. Conversely, listening closely, leaning toward the patient during conversation, and smiling improves the communication experience. When used appropriately, smiles are almost universally accepted as a gesture of good will and a means of establishing a friendly rapport.

Proxemics

Proxemics is the term used to describe the **spatial** relationships (physical closeness) tolerated by most people. How near or far we place ourselves from others transmits strong messages (Box 1-4). North Americans usually consider the space within approximately 3 feet as personal space, although this varies among individuals. This space also varies greatly with our relationship to those around us—from a small space for close family members to a wider space for strangers. Stress levels rise significantly and measurably when personal space is invaded without permission.

Box **1-4   Physical Reactions in Proxemics**

Think about how you react as you stand in a line or ride in an elevator. Americans usually step back when a stranger, or even an acquaintance without permission, steps into our personal space. If personal space is reduced for too long, symptoms of stress increase. These include a rise in blood pressure and heart rate, an increase in respirations, and feelings of panic. For the patient who is already stressed by illness or worry, it is important that we restore personal space as soon as possible after care.

In the medical setting, our physical distance from patients may be affected by odors, such as poor physical or dental hygiene, decay, or odors associated with certain illnesses. Patients may be upset by smells in the medical setting, such as disinfectants and medicinal scents, particularly if they bring back unpleasant memories of previous medical experiences. Use caution with your own hygiene. Patients may object to the smell of cigarettes or food on you and your clothing and may be uncomfortable with the perfume or body lotion that smells good to you. All of these factors have an impact on interaction with patients in the close-up, hands-on, medical environment.

In certain cases, physical distance may be limited for infection control. For example, if your patient has a communicable disease, direct contact may be limited. Many communicable diseases require physical barriers, such as masks and gloves, which may interfere with facial expressions and with using touch as a communication tool. Methods for overcoming these communication barriers are covered later in Chapter 2, "Challenges to Communication."

Even with our highly technological medical environment, we usually need to enter patients' personal space to deliver care. Because some people are uncomfortable when their personal space is invaded, and our patients are already stressed, it is important to develop a therapeutic rapport early in the relationship. Approach patients in a confident and professional manner, introduce yourself, and tell them what you plan to do. Explain the purpose of each step of the procedure. If patients shrink away or act fearful, reassure them that you will allow them to direct the interaction, and that you will stop at any point they indicate discomfort. Patients have a right to self-determination and may accept or refuse any contact or treatment if they choose. Patients do not have to submit to an invasion of their space. Back away when you are finished, unless patients signal a need for closeness. Be alert to positive or negative signs that let you know the patient accepts you in his space. Signs of fear and increased stress usually indicate patients are uncomfortable and that you need to step back; leaning in your direction and maintaining eye contact may mean that they prefer that you offer comfort by staying near. These actions, and a professional attitude, help relieve patients' anxiety regarding care and the manner in which it is provided. Remember, it is important to allow patients to make decisions regarding their personal space and to respect their preferences.

Touch as a Communication Tool

Proxemics, and the concept of spatial relationships, includes touch. Touch is required for procedures related to health care. You may use touch with patients to indicate emotional support or to show concern. There is no better way to demonstrate caring and compassion to those who are "starved" for contact. Remember that some elderly patients are not touched

Box **1-5**   **Therapeutic Touch**

Touch as a means of healing has a long and **credible** history. Divine touch is recorded in most of the world's religions. In medieval Europe and England, the "king's touch" was thought to cure many illnesses. Sick people lined the roadways when the royal procession was scheduled to pass, hoping to touch the hem of the king's robe, or, if one was lucky, to have the king actually reach out and touch a hand or face. It did not seem to matter that the cure rate was understandably extremely low.

We no longer believe in the "king's touch," of course, but we do know that babies are more likely to die if they are not held and stroked, and that the elderly have measurably decreased levels of stress and pain if they are stroked and touched gently. Today, the ancient healing practices of touch (Reiki) and therapeutic **massage** are gaining favor in holistic medical practices. The theory holds that the body produces life energy, or "prana." When patients feel prana through touch, healing energy is produced. This energy provides emotional, physical, and spiritual comfort. Some hospitals and practices use these techniques to reduce pain and promote wound healing. A simple, caring touch may be the most therapeutic procedure you can perform for any patient.

by anyone for long periods of time, which increases their feeling of isolation when their hearing and vision are failing and moves them further away from social interaction. Although some patients welcome a caring touch, others may not be comfortable with physical contact. Touch is cultural; some patients prefer that you not touch them except for treatment purposes. Many feel that touch in a medical setting signals that something unpleasant is about to happen. If you feel the patient will be receptive, offer a comforting touch when nothing invasive or painful is planned.

There is an increased need to use therapeutic touch with a warm and caring hand in our technologically advanced medical setting. However, before using touch as a means of showing concern and compassion, determine by watching the patient whether your touch is welcome. Without permission being granted, touching implies a certain intimacy and establishes power to the one who is touching over the one who is touched. Patients may feel that you will withhold your care and concern if they are honest about not wishing to be touched except for therapeutic care. In certain situations, an unwelcome touch may be considered assault. Therefore, either implied or explicit permission must be granted. For instance, a patient who responds to your comforting touch by covering your hand with hers or by leaning toward you, welcomes your touch; conversely, a patient who stiffens, leans away from you or crosses her arms and legs is sending messages that your touch is not welcome (Box 1-5).

STARTING OFF RIGHT

How you approach your patients gives them clues to observe about you, just as you are observing them. They know quickly how professional you are by your poise, your physical appearance, and your actions. They hope that you will work for their trust and confidence, and that if you do not have answers to all of the questions, you can search for the answers together.

Patients frequently have preformed opinions of health care workers that may interfere with establishing an initial rapport. There are those who think all health care professionals except the physician are there to fill a servant-like role, and these people will look down on anyone other than the physician. There are also those who are in awe of all health care professionals and expect you to know all of the answers. Work for a balance in your interaction with both types of patients; do not be either overly friendly or distant and inaccessible. Stress that we are in the health care field for our patients but that our scope of practice does not give any of us all of the answers. Speak respectfully and maintain your professionalism during all interactions to help establish and maintain positive patient relationships.

Addressing Your Patient

As you greet your patients, use a proper form of address, for example, "Mr. Green, how are you today?" or "How may we help you, Mrs. Brown?" Never address a patient by his or her first name unless requested to do so by the patient, and never use pet names, such as "Honey" or "Sweetie." Children, of course, or those younger than you will not expect to be addressed by their surname, but patients older than you should be treated with the respect that we show by using surnames. Certain ethnic cultures will be offended by familiarity that we see as being friendly. Patients who insist on communicating with you on a first-name basis may not understand the therapeutic nature of the patient/health care professional relationship. This is not a friendship, though you may be genuinely fond of your patients; this is a professional relationship. It may be flattering to have patients try to establish a more personal relationship, but this will interfere with your ability to administer proper care. Try to determine why the patient needs to be addressed on a personal level and wants to move the relationship to a friendship, but maintain your professional distance.

Never refer to your patient as a medical condition, for example, "the fracture in the treatment room" or "the post-op in Room 3." Patients are understandably stressed and anxious in the health care setting and are sensitive to everything they see and hear (or overhear). If you refer to patients simply as a medical condition, anyone who overhears you will presume you do not care for your patients as individuals.

Maintaining a Professional Distance

Interaction and communication are affected by our emotional involvement with others. For instance, we interact differently with our parents, our significant other, our children, and our friends, and each interaction is more intimate on many levels than our response to acquaintances and persons in the workplace. Communication and interaction in the health care setting must be conducted on a level that allows us to work closely with patients, observe their care and condition effectively, and provide opportunities for patient teaching. Professional distance allows us to work with patients while maintaining a therapeutic relationship. The focus must be on patients, not on our concerns; never share confidences with patients about your personal life that might shift the dynamics of the relationship to a more personal level. Patients have their own concerns and should not be burdened with ours. If your patient tries to engage in a personal exchange, briefly, politely, and truthfully answer just that question—never answer rudely—but quickly and firmly turn the topic back to health care. If you find yourself trying to establish friendships with patients, step back and determine why you are searching for friendship among your patients, rather than in a more proper social environment. Recognize that it would be extremely difficult to give effective care to a friend, and search for your friends outside of the medical setting.

Sympathy and Empathy

Closely linked to the concept of professional distance are the expressions of **sympathy** and **empathy**. Sympathy implies that you care and that you feel pity and compassion for the feelings of another; empathy more closely means identifying with and understanding another person on a deeper level. In other words, sympathy usually means feeling sorry for someone. Sympathy does not require that we identify with the patient and is usually an expression of sharing the pain but may not result in efforts to relieve the suffering. Empathy means understanding at a deep level what the patient feels and involves a deep need to relieve the concern, usually because we, as individuals, have experienced the same or very similar circumstances.

When we empathize, we suspend our own perceptions and, at least for a time, try to feel what the patient feels. We may feel sorry for or sympathize with a patient who is dying and may distance ourselves. When we empathize, we imagine how it would feel to *be* the patient and do all in our power to provide comfort and care because we *almost* know how he feels. To achieve or develop an empathetic character, set aside preconceptions and open your mind to personal differences and perceptions. We each react differently to pain, loss, sickness, and suffering. We do not have to change our firmly held beliefs and values to genuinely care for our patients, but we must understand that differences do exist and work around these differences.

We must be sincerely committed to the need to relieve suffering to put ourselves in the position of caring. Sharing a patient's suffering may open us to pain, but the goal of excellence in health care is worth the challenge. Empathizing helps us recognize a patient's fear and discomfort so that we do everything possible to provide support and reassurance.

KEEPING COMMUNICATION ON TRACK

If your interaction with the patient did not establish a therapeutic relationship, learn from it for the future. Avoid establishing a dependent relationship with the patient; your goal, and his, should be his independence and self-care. He should be free and competent to make proper health care choices and perform his own care independent of your skills. You must have a strong self-concept and be able to let go of your need to encourage the patient's dependence on you. Independence in health care is the purpose of therapeutic interaction.

If problems developed during your communication and your efforts to help the patient were not effective, mentally review the exchange. What could you have done differently? Were there factors in the interaction that blocked the communication flow, or disrupted the communication agreement with the patient? Or did you form a bond that was not appropriate for proper health care?

To establish a better working relationship or rapport with the patient, try these suggestions at each contact:

- Before you begin, know the goal of the communication—that is, asking about current concerns, offering educational material, transferring information—but be flexible. The patient may have other needs that you discover only after the exchange has begun.
- Avoid clichéd statements. "You'll be just fine" sounds false, diminishes the patient's concerns, and may sound suspiciously like a guarantee, which could lead to legal action.

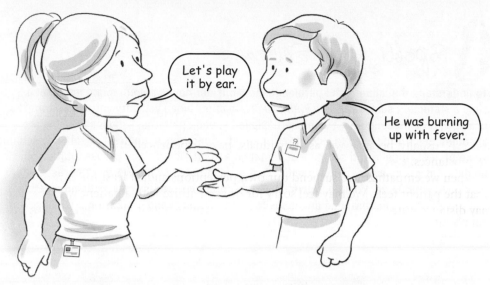

Figure 1-4

- Do not offer false reassurance. Explain the health care plan and its possible benefits but do not offer unrealistic hope. Again, this may seem to the patient to promise that he will improve, when this may not be the case.
- Avoid using idioms. An **idiom** is a well-known phrase or sentence with a meaning completely different from its literal translation. These include sayings such as, "Let's play it by ear," or "He was burning up with fever." These do not translate well to patients who use English as a second language (Fig. 1-4).
- If patients need to talk about themselves and their situation, do not change the subject immediately, even to redirect it to the topic at hand. You may discover issues that are affecting their health and that need attention. You might miss these concerns with tightly focused questioning. However, if patients begin to ramble too far from the need for health care, gently nudge them toward the current problem.
- Do not moralize. It is not our place to impose our values on our patients. Try to understand patients even if you do not agree.
- Avoid leading questions that suggest the answer that you want, such as, "You are taking your medicine, aren't you?" Many patients want to agree with you and will give you an answer they think you expect.
- Do not cue patients by your facial expressions or other kinesics. If they sense that the direction of the message is uncomfortable for you, they may stop trying to communicate.
- Control your tone of voice to convey sincerity and compassion without overdoing it. Sugary, flowery tones and language sound false (see Spotlight on Success box).
- Allow patients to make suggestions for their care; they know their situation better than you and may have good ideas. If you have self-esteem and a solid self-concept, you should not be threatened by changes in health care plans to meet your patients' needs.

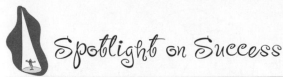

Spotlight on Success

To understand the influence of paralanguage, consider how a patient might interpret a simple statement such as *"I'll be with you in a minute"* when you vary your voice tone. For example, an impatient tone—with short, clipped speech patterns—implies that you are impatient and far too busy to listen to the patient's concerns. In contrast, a soft, low-pitched voice projects a calm and soothing acceptance and attitude. Try the phrase with emphasis on different words and see how communication is affected by the words or phrases you choose to emphasize. Using paralanguage appropriately increases your communication skills in all areas of interaction and leads to better personal and professional success and satisfaction.

- Sequence your questions from less complex or general, to more complex and specific. "How are you today?" should progress to questions such as "Can you describe the problem?" (This is covered in Chapter 3, "Gathering Information.")
- If you cannot answer a question, be truthful. You will be more credible and professional for admitting that you do not have all of the answers than if you try to respond to a question for which you have no answer.

Observing these factors in communication and genuinely caring for your patients should result in relationships that lead to better health and that challenge and reward you as a professional.

 ### Taking the Chapter to Work

Now, let's meet Jessica and see how she has applied this chapter information in the workplace.

Jessica is working in a family practice office. She has just walked a young female patient into an examination room. The patient is 15 years old and has an appointment for a Pap test and gynecological examination. While Jessica takes the patient's blood pressure and pulse, she notices that the patient does not maintain eye contact and is fidgeting and squirming in the chair. Jessica recognizes these kinesics as possible signs of anxiety and nervousness. To help alleviate these feelings, Jessica sits down in a chair next to the patient and begins to communicate with her. Jessica uses touch as a soothing technique. After a few minutes, the patient appears less anxious. Jessica knows that many patients are anxious about undressing, so she decides to have the patient stay dressed and sit in the chair until the physician comes in to talk to her. Jessica communicates her observations to the physician. Working as a team, they are able to reassure the patient and complete the examination without problems. The outcome of this situation would have been very different if Jessica had ignored or not noticed these signs.

B e y o n d the Classroom Exercises

Your Assignment Board:

The following exercises will help you use your new knowledge. Place a check beside the assignments your instructor has given you. When you have completed the assignment, place a check in the completed column.

		Assigned	*Completed*
Checking Your Comprehension	(Textbook)	❏	❏
Expanding Critical Thinking	(Textbook)	❏	❏
Communication Surfer Exercises	(Textbook and Internet)	❏	❏
Communication Tree Branch #1	(CD-ROM)	❏	❏
Voice Mail Message #1	(CD-ROM)	❏	❏

 ## Checking Your Comprehension

Write a brief answer for each of the following assignments.
1. Explain the three steps to effective communication.
2. List five of your responsibilities in the communication process.
3. List four of your patient's responsibilities in the communication process.
4. Define and compare the terms *kinesics* and *proxemics*. Give two examples of each.
5. How does *sympathy* differ from *empathy*? Which one offers more help to patients and why?
6. What is meant by the phrase *therapeutic touch*? How is touch used in the medical profession?

 ## Communication Surfer Exercises

1. Using a search engine, type in the term *HIPAA*. How many sites did you find? Narrow your sites to find the official government website. What types of communication violations could cause you to be fined? Either print the webpage information or write a list of potential communication violations.
2. Search the Internet and find a site illustrating current news articles. By looking at only the illustrations, describe what the facial expressions are communicating. Print six different pictures or clips and write a headline or description for each.
3. Hint: Refer to Figure 1-3 for illustrations of various facial expressions.
Using a search engine, type in the word *idiom*. Print a list of commonly used idioms. How many of these do you use in everyday communication? Choose five commonly used idioms and describe how they can be misunderstood.

Expanding Critical Thinking

1. Consider these situations:
   a. You have explained to Mr. Brown how to collect a first voided specimen for tomorrow.

   Response: You receive a stool specimen in the urine container.

   Why do you think Mr. Brown misunderstood your instructions? Was the message received as intended? Was the message in a form he could interpret? How could you have made sure that he understood? How should you respond to him when he presents you with the wrong specimen? Whose fault is it that he misunderstood?

   b. Mrs. Simmons is in a moderately advanced stage of Alzheimer's disease and has very limited responses to conversation and stimulus. You know, however, that you must talk to her as if she understands, as you would with any patient. You explain to her what you must do for her at each step of the procedure.

   Response A. Her eyes follow your movements with mild interest, but she makes no other response.

   Response B. You receive no response from her throughout the procedure, even to fairly unpleasant stimuli.

   Which component of the communication flow is missing in Response B? Is more than one component missing? Can the response in Response A be considered verification that she received your message?

2. List 10 examples of nonverbal communication you experienced today. Examples may include a smile from a friend, a message on a T-shirt, a yawn from your spouse. Next to each of these items, indicate the following:
   a. Did you respond positively or negatively to the communication?
   b. Do you think the sender of the message intended for you to have that response?

3. Considering proxemics, should there be a difference between the professional distances of men to men, women to men, women to women? How do you feel when a male doctor stands close to you? Or a female doctor? Are you comfortable standing close to the opposite sex in a professional situation? How do you seal yourself off in a public place—with books, bags, folded arms, etc? Do you sit in the same seat each class session? Do you look for a seat near or far from other students?

4. Body language and nonverbal cues carry as many messages as the spoken word. Read the following and identify the cues the person is sending, then answer the accompanying questions. "Fie, fie upon her! There's language in her eyes, her cheek, her lip. Nay, her foot speaks; her wanton spirits look at every joint and motive in her body." (William Shakespeare in "Troilus and Cressida")
   a. How has communication changed in the past 400 years? 100 years?
   b. How do you think it will changed in the next 400 years? 100 years?
   c. What do you think Shakespeare meant by the above description?
   d. Rewrite the description in today's terms.

Expanding Critical Thinking—Cont'd

5. List five common idioms that you hear or say frequently. Write the literal meaning and then the intended meaning. Draw a picture or cartoon illustrating the idiom.

6. Do you consider yourself a positive or a negative personality? Name five of your positive and five of your negative traits. Have a family member or good friend make a list for you and compare the two.

7. Write a brief paragraph describing how you think others see you.

8. List ways to increase your self-esteem. Now list ways to increase someone else's self-esteem.

9. Plan an initial interaction as you get to know the following patients. What will you talk about to establish rapport?
   a. An elderly widower who lives alone with no close family.
   b. An HIV-positive former drug addict who has been drug free for more than a year.
   c. An HIV-positive prostitute in the early stages of the full-blown syndrome.
   d. A young mother of four who suspects she is pregnant again and does not want another child.
   e. A 5-year-old Hispanic boy who speaks very little English and is clinging to his mother who speaks almost no English.
   f. A 45-year-old woman whose latest breast biopsy indicates that her cancer has returned.

2

CHALLENGES TO COMMUNICATION: OVERCOMING THE BARRIERS

LEARNING OBJECTIVES

Upon successfully completing this chapter, you will be able to:

- Explain how barriers to communication interfere with establishing rapport.
- Describe how differences in cultural perspectives affect communication and explain methods to prevent this barrier.
- List ways to communicate with patients for whom English is a second language.
- Explain how to approach communication with patients who have impairments in hearing, vision, language, or cognition or who are too ill to communicate.
- Give examples of how stress and anger interfere with communication and how to relieve the situation.
- Give examples of age-related barriers and list ways to work within the age groups.
- Explain how personal biases interfere with interaction and list ways to overcome the barriers.

KEY TERMS

Amulet	Cohesive	Inflection
Anacusis	Cultural imposition	Interdependent
Appease, appeased	Culture	Matriarchal
Assimilate, assimilation	Discriminate, discrimination	Patriarchal
Autonomy	Escalate	Presbycusis
Belligerence, belligerent	Ethnic, ethnicity	Respite
Bias	Impedance	Subjective

Test Your Communication IQ

Before reading this chapter, complete this short self-assessment test. Decide which statements are true and which are false.

1. Patients who do not ask for clarification following a lengthy explanation may feel embarrassed or intimidated by health care professionals.
2. Cultural rituals give specific groups their identity and promote a cohesive environment.
3. Americans tend to be an interdependent society.
4. In a patriarchal society, the oldest female makes all of the decisions.
5. A flat speech pattern with little inflection may indicate a hearing impairment.
6. Visual impairments may interfere with your ability to communicate effectively with a patient.
7. Patients who are acutely ill often wish to engage in lengthy discussions about their medical condition in the hope that their symptoms can be eliminated.
8. A child's developmental stage will always regress during an illness.

Results

Statements one, two, five, and six are true; all other statements are false. How did you do? Read the chapter to learn more about these topics.

CHALLENGES TO COMMUNICATION

Communicating is usually easy when patients are your same sex, about your same age, from roughly the same socioeconomic and educational background, and with an approximately equal degree of health. Having similar cultural and life-experience background also helps. However, even if you and your patient have many life factors in common, it is not likely that you share the same degree of health unless the patient needs nothing more today than a routine physical examination. In most instances, you and your patients come together with very different values, views, and perspectives. In medical situations, patients and caregivers are usually too stressed to put aside their concerns and make the extra effort to understand and communicate with you; it is your responsibility to adapt your communication style to the needs of each situation.

In this chapter, we cover many obvious barriers to communication, but in practice, other barriers are less apparent and may block an exchange as abruptly as factors that we recognize quickly, such as age and language. Careful health care professionals work to avoid controllable barriers. The types of questions suggested below should help you identify less obvious factors before they interfere with communication.

• Have you evaluated the patient's understanding and level of education to determine how to focus the interaction? Are you speaking above or below the patient's comprehension? Are you sure your message is clearly stated and appropriate for the patient?
• Are you and the patient ready to communicate? Is she confused, stressed, or too ill today? Are you distracted, rushed, or not prepared for the interaction?
• Does the patient feel pressured? Have your nonverbal cues communicated your lack of time and patience? Have you given him time to organize his thoughts or are you rushing through the exchange?

- Does the environment encourage a private, confidential exchange? Is it noisy? Are interruptions a problem? Are others coming and going? Is the room uncomfortable? Is concentration difficult because it is too warm or too cool for comfort?
- Does the patient feel confident to confide in you? Does she feel that her information is safe with you? Have you established an appropriate rapport?

Observe patients during any exchange for signs that communication barriers are developing. Some patients feel that it must be their fault if they cannot understand you and are reluctant to ask you to slow down or explain something again. Patients who keep trying to change the subject or who laugh inappropriately may be uncomfortable or embarrassed by the topic. Those who have no questions may not have grasped what you said and may be reluctant to ask for clarification. A good, respectful rapport helps patients feel comfortable to ask you or tell you whatever is on their mind.

Avoidable Barriers to Communication

Barriers that should never become an issue in a therapeutic relationship, and are totally under your control, include the following:

- Clichéd statements: "Look on the bright side." "It could have been worse." These overused statements make patients feel they are not valued as individuals with unique concerns.
- Contradicting: "It could not have happened that way." "Are you sure of what you are saying?" Contradicting implies the patient is not being truthful. If you suspect that what you are hearing is less than the truth, carefully restate your questions for more reliable information. (See Chapter 3, "Gathering Information," for additional discussion.)
- Criticizing: "You know you should have called us as soon as this happened." Critical statements make patients feel guilty and may build a defensive barrier.
- Ridiculing: "That was a dumb thing to do." As with criticizing, a response such as this stops communication immediately.
- Sarcasm: "Oh, great! This is just what you need." Sarcasm states one thing but implies the opposite. These statements made in a sarcastic tone may be misunderstood, especially if your patient speaks English as a second language. This particular example is confusing since whatever the concern was in this case was certainly not something the patient felt he needed.
- Indifference: Patients feel that you do not value their concerns if they suspect you are not focused on communicating. Watch your nonverbal cues and kinesics to keep the channels of communication open. These cues and kinesics include glancing at your watch, yawning, or staring off in the distance while the patient is talking.
- Lecturing or offering unsolicited advice: "You know you shouldn't be smoking." "Why aren't you watching your diet?" Do not confuse lecturing with patient education. Lecturing serves no purpose except to scold the patient; patient education can save his life.

The communication barriers listed above all have negative effects and are committed intentionally or at least without proper concern for the patient's feelings. These are barriers you can control and avoid. They will stop therapeutic interaction in an instant and make it hard to reestablish a workable rapport.

A less negative but still controllable barrier response involves inexact language. Much of what we say does not translate well for those for whom English is a second language. Even English-speaking patients may have trouble with concepts such as large/small, fast/slow, warm/hot. For example, what may look like a small amount of blood to us may seem large to the patient who is bleeding. Try to be as exact as possible regarding **subjective** terms, such as those listed above, and use examples that are less personal or open to interpretation. Examples such as, "A spot of blood this size," with a demonstration may be more appropriate. Other examples include, "If your pulse goes above this number, give us a call," or "If your peak flow does not reach this level, let us know." Using terms that patients can identify cuts down on confusion.

Idioms are a common form of inexact language that block communication. We take these terms for granted; they add color, humor, and description to our conversations. However, patients may not understand what they mean. Think of times you have used idioms such as those illustrated in Figure 2-1, and how patients may misunderstand or be understandably confused by a common idiom.

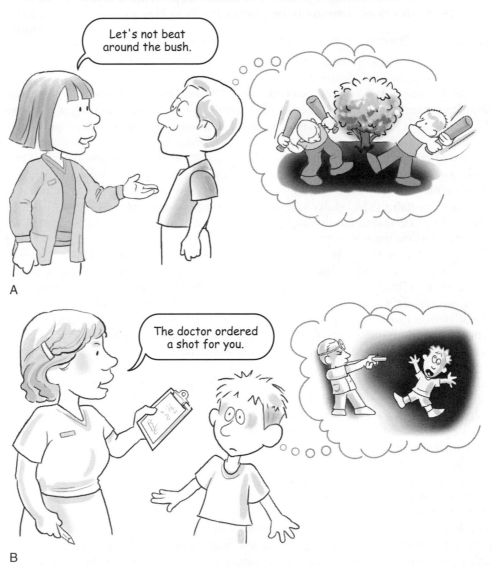

Figure 2-1

The barriers, or challenges, listed through the rest of the chapter may be apparent early in an interaction. Plan carefully for possible responses to potential barriers before you begin working with patients to establish an appropriate rapport and to demonstrate professionalism.

CULTURAL CHALLENGES

Cultures are divided and defined by the knowledge, values, beliefs, and rules that are part of the groups to which we belong. Culture is taught to us by our caregivers from birth, shared by our group, formed by our geographical environment, and constantly changing to meet the needs of our community. Our cultural rituals give our group its identity and help keep it united and **cohesive** (staying together). Our culture helps us make decisions and respond to most of the situations common to our group. It tells us how to interact, react, feel, and behave. These traditions guide our thinking and our behavior in such a deeply ingrained and unconscious manner that we may not even be aware of their influence.

Culture sets the standards for such perceptions as the measures of success, the ideals of beauty, and personal interactions, such as group interdependence versus self-reliance. For example, success to Americans is usually financial independence, beauty is usually tall and thin, and we value independence, rather than depending on others to help us. These cultural perceptions affect every aspect of our lives but may not be shared by other groups. Collective or **interdependent** cultures are more focused on their family and their group; Americans tend to be more individualistic or independent. Interdependent societies rely on the collective wisdom of the group to make decisions, even those affecting health; we tend to think and decide for ourselves. We work hard to maintain our independence; interdependent societies work equally as hard to maintain group unity. Our culture makes sense to us and works for us but may not be realistic for all of our patients. Presuming that everyone should feel and act as we do, and imposing our behaviors on others, is called **cultural imposition**. Refusing to recognize differences is called cultural blindness. In health care, we tend to practice cultural blindness when we expect all patients to react the same in every situation, regardless of traditions and needs. For example, when we refuse or neglect to consider the nontraditional healing methods of another culture, we are guilty of cultural blindness. If we impose our views on the patient who is reluctant to go against his society's values, we are guilty of cultural imposition. In the health care field, such attitudes drive away patients who need our care. This obviously is not therapeutic communication.

Culture also determines how patients view illness versus wellness, how they react to pain, how they feel about the health care profession versus folk or natural healers, whether they feel they have control over their health, and whether they will follow health care directives contrary to their culture. Since our patient population is culturally diverse, we must learn as much as possible about their needs and traditions before the health care encounter. When we learn about other cultures, we tend to set aside our prejudices based on our own ignorance. Look at your own culture and recognize how important your place in your community is to you. When you can do this objectively, you will be more aware of how alike we all are and will be much more tolerant of differences.

All areas of the country have an intermingling of many cultures, each practicing traditions that affect health and health care compliance. Many of our patients hold onto their native traditions rather than following a health care plan that seems strange to them, particularly if it contradicts their religion or values. Many cultures are more afraid of social rejection than they are of illness. For example, if a woman's value to the family depends on her ability to conceive, she is not likely to agree to a hysterectomy regardless of the consequences to her health. If socializing within the culture depends on large family meals with many heavy dishes, cutting down on fats and calories may be an insult to the family and its traditions. Factors such as these should influence how we approach communication and patient education with cultures other than our own. Imposing our expectations and trying to change culture-based patterns of behavior increases the patient's stress level. It takes great tact and diplomacy to direct the patient to healthful life choices if these choices directly oppose cultural traditions.

Within each large culture, such as here in America, are many subcultures (Box 2-1). For instance, North versus South, white collar versus blue collar, young versus old, and so forth, and each defines the behaviors expected of its members.

The subcultures listed in Box 2-1 are almost as broad as the major cultures. Within any of these subcultures are also further divisions, such as provinces of China, Native American tribes, and African-American ancestries spread through many regions. All of these factors affect health care based on physical characteristics, dietary habits, genetic heritage, and religious practices. To relate to the groups present in your community, learn as much as you can about the cultures, beliefs, practices, and customary diet. Rather than trying to change these beliefs and customs, try to work within the cultural traditions. If the physician feels that the patient's cultural practices are affecting his health, it is the physician's responsibility to discuss this with the patient.

Suggestions for interacting with cultures different from our own usually involve common sense, good manners, and a high tolerance for differences, such as the following:
- Learn as much as possible about the cultures represented in your area. See these differences as an opportunity to grow in cultural understanding.
- Stress the things that most cultures have in common and accept the differences.

Box 2-1   Subcultures

We tend to think of geographical or national areas as having just one culture within the borders. When we consider the many different nationalities and ethnic groups in our own nation, we realize others have just as many intermingled cultural groups as we do. All of these groups practice traditions that may be important to consider in health care.

Subcultures you may see in your medical practice include the following:
- Anglo-American: this designation includes western European countries such as England, France, and Germany.
- African-American: ancestry from any of the countries within the African subcontinent.
- Latino: includes Puerto Rico, Cuba, Mexico, and South and Central America. The term Chicano generally refers to Mexican descent and Hispanic to other Spanish-speaking ancestry.
- Asian-American: countries of origin or ancestry include China, Japan, Korea, The Philippines, Thailand, Vietnam.
- Native American: includes all tribes of American Indians, including Eskimos and Aleuts.
- Eastern European: Russian, Polish, Serbian.
- Middle Eastern: includes Arabic, Pakistani, Iranian, Iraqi, and Israeli.

- Always assume that patients prefer that you use the family name unless you are given expressed permission to use a given name. This is true of all patients, but is especially important in other cultures.
- Encourage patients to talk about their illnesses and look for areas of misunderstanding between cultural beliefs and the current diagnosis.
- Look for confusion and fear; watch for cues and respond with compassion. Do not ignore culture-based anxiety. Talk to your patients and explain why and how the health care directives help recovery.
- Evaluate nonverbal communication by observing proxemics, kinesics, and other cues (see Chapter 1, "Introduction to Communication"). They may be very different from yours.
- Treat all patients with respect, concern, and compassion. Try to learn what it is about this illness that this patient sees as most important. It may be different from your reaction to the same illness.
- Determine what is important in this culture. What are the religious doctrines and food rituals? How do persons in this culture respond to pain? What is the general level of hygiene?
- Find out who makes the decisions. In **matriarchal** societies, the oldest female makes all decisions; in **patriarchal** societies, it is the oldest male relative. This patient may not consent to treatment without consulting the authority figure in the group.
- Be aware that the dominant authority figure in this patient's group may accompany the patient and may be the one to whom you direct questions and give instructions. The patient may not be allowed to respond or make decisions without this person's permission.
- Recognize that other societies are not as time-sensitive as Americans. A 10:00 a.m. appointment may mean any time in the morning, or even tomorrow. Your exasperation will not change this behavior, but your understanding will change your exasperation.
- Understand that certain cultures avoid eye contact as a matter of respect. Many Asian populations, Native Americans, Arabs, and certain Hispanic groups consider it rude and disrespectful to meet your eyes. For example, Latino women are taught that downcast eyes are a proper response to authority. This is not avoidance; this is tradition.
- Recognize that many cultures are less likely than most Americans to "get to the point." They may see a brief, exact response as abrupt or rude. Rather than "yes/no" or other brief answers, they may give elaborate responses to avoid appearing rude.
- Be aware that not expressing pain or illness may be a cultural response. Look for incongruent messages. If the patient appears ill or in pain but denies it, he may feel he cannot acknowledge what he sees as weakness. The outward appearance of strength may be his cultural tradition.
- Acknowledge that many cultures are intensely involved with the supernatural and may believe that spirits, hexes, and the like cause illness. In these cultures, the supernatural must be **appeased** (soothed or satisfied) before healing can begin (Box 2-2).
- Incorporate the patient's folk remedies into treatment if at all possible. In fact, you should ask if he or she has consulted a folk healer. If the answer is "yes," try to determine what therapies the patient is using.
- Learn about the many current medicines and treatments that started as folk or herbal remedies. Talk with your physician about those the patient is using. It may be possible to incorporate them into standard treatment.
- Discuss the health care directives to determine whether these will separate the patient from the group's rituals and traditions. If this happens, you cannot realistically expect compliance.

Box **2-2** Cultural Healers

Many ethnic societies have long histories with folk or cultural healers. These include the Indian shaman, the Korean mansin, the Haitian mambo, the African sangona, the Chinese wu, and the Spanish curandera. To these societies, our medicine is considered alternative medicine.

Cultures that depend on these healers feel they have many advantages over traditional medicine, including those listed below:

- They speak the same language, live in the same environment, and understand the cultural traditions.
- The society may believe the healer is endowed with special powers to heal, perhaps by divine assignment.
- They are usually less expensive. Many trade in barter, or an exchange of goods, such as food or other items.
- While our medical profession relies on technology to determine the cause of illness, healers seem to know instinctively. Most are excellent at reading cues and may have the advantage of more personal knowledge of the patient's history and current situation.
- They are more accessible and understand the patient's needs in a personal and cultural perspective.

Do not try to change patients' beliefs in traditional healers; this only adds to the stress of illness. If at all possible, the best course is to include as many cultural beliefs and traditions as is reasonable into the patient's treatment plan.

- Be aware of the preferred diet. New Food Guide Pyramids are adapted to many ethnic diets. These are covered in Chapter 5, "Communicating Wellness."
- If you must impose on the patient's culture by entering private space or by asking probing questions that make patients uncomfortable, apologize and explain why this is necessary.

Other Cultural Barriers

We are usually aware of national and **ethnic** cultural differences, but there are other cultures within our society, such as wealth versus poverty, male versus female, and youth versus age. Any of these individual differences can interfere with understanding and rapport.

Wealth versus poverty has far-reaching health care significance and is one of the most difficult barriers to overcome. Since most health care workers are middle class, the cultures at opposite ends of the socioeconomic spectrum are almost as alien as those from distant countries. For example, wealthier patients have better access to health care and generally consult health care providers much earlier than patients who have no permanent physician and who rely on emergency room physicians. The underprivileged are less likely to be well educated and may not understand what they hear in the medical setting. With less self-esteem and self-worth, they are less likely to ask for clarification about anything they do not understand. Wealthy people are usually very concerned with wellness and practice consistent preventive care. Poor people only "fix it" when it is too "broken" to tolerate, since needs other than wellness are far more important, such as a place to live and food to eat (see Chapter 4, "Educating Patients" for discussion of Maslow's hierarchy). Wealthy people may be treated better by health care professionals than the underprivileged because of issues such as hygiene, pre-sumed compliance, background knowledge of the presenting disorder, and, unfortunately, ability to pay for care. With so many stressors, disadvantaged patients are more likely than wealthy patients to use inappropriate coping mechanisms, such as substance abuse and domestic violence, although neither group is immune to these problems. Poor patients are more likely to see the health care worker as well educated; wealthy patients may see you as someone hired to serve them. If you can think of poverty and wealth as simply other cultures, each with its own language and customs, you will be better able to interact with both groups.

Male culture versus female culture also may be significant. Stereotypically, many men are taught to be strong about pain, to "tough it out," and to see illness as weakness. Conversely, when they do admit to illness, some men regress and expect to be comforted. (Regression as a coping mechanism is covered in Chapter 5, "Communicating Wellness.") Women, if they have the luxury to do so, may have been taught that illness and weakness are acceptable female reactions. For many generations, women were expected to "swoon" (faint) and actu-ally had "fainting couches" to sink into at the first sight or mention of anything unpleasant. Of course, those who had the luxury of swooning were usually wealthy; there is no record that ladies' maids were allowed to swoon. Since women as a group have been conditioned by society to be more vocal about their feelings, they frequently are seen as complainers.

Youth versus age as a communication challenge is covered later in this chapter. As we will discuss, life stages present barriers unique to each group.

LANGUAGE BARRIERS

In any communication exchange, the sender is responsible for transmitting the message in a form the receiver can understand, and the receiver is responsible for making an effort to interpret the message as it was intended. The entire message includes all of the cues we have discussed, such as paralanguage, kinesics, and so on. As we have seen, this is difficult, even when both participants speak the same language and use somewhat the same nonverbal cues. Imagine then how hard it is to communicate with different cultural expectations and different languages.

When you interact with patients who speak either no English or limited English, you must be especially careful to encourage communication and to respond to the patient's needs. Your best and most therapeutic response is to learn the dominant cultural languages in your area. If this is not practical, and you are not able to learn even a few phrases appropriate to your specialty, other methods listed below help make messages reasonably clear.

In the absence of a common language, you may use an interpreter. If someone on staff is fluent in the patient's language, this may be the best solution. Health care professionals will know how to pursue a line of questioning and can determine what medical information is needed in different situations. On the other hand, family members may have the advantage of knowing the patient's history and can anticipate responses, which may save time and frus-tration. This may not be the best solution, however, when the patient is uncomfortable shar-ing information through a family member, and where confidentiality is an issue.

Interpreters can be recruited from places of worship and ethnic organizations. These vol-unteers are eager to help with cultural **assimilation**, or acceptance into the adopted com-munity, and usually have interpreters of different age groups for both sexes. Ideally, interpreters of the same sex and near the patient's age work best, since some cultures forbid exchanges of intimate information between sexes. Although it may not be the best solution, interpreters are also available by phone in certain situations. If no interpreter is available, or time is too limited to recruit someone, a phrase book or flash cards may help, presuming the patient is literate in his own language. Pictures or sketches related to medical questions can be used if the patient is a nonreader. Several picture dictionary aids are available to show procedures and ask questions in a tasteful manner for patients who are nonreaders. Demonstration and pantomime may work also, but medical situations may be hard to translate into action.

Once you have in place a means of communication, the following guidelines make the exchange more productive:

- When using an interpreter, face both the interpreter and the patient so they can see you and read your communication cues. In this position, you will see both participants and can read their cues as they read yours. Patients need to see your face and may understand more English than they speak. In this position, patients may be able to participate in the exchange.
- Use your normal tone of voice. Shouting will not make your words easier to understand and may be seen as anger in some cultures.
- Follow the Rule of Fives used for many of the communication barriers that we will discuss in this chapter: sentences no longer than five words, words of no more than five letters. Short sentences and short words are easier to translate.
- Keep the exchange simple. For example, ask if the patient has pain, terms such as "discomfort" may be harder to translate.
- Ask as many "yes" or "no" questions as possible without limiting the scope of answers. Many patients understand English better than they speak it, and it helps patients feel they are contributing when they can respond even if they do not speak the language well enough to form an extended answer.
- Ask one question at a time and rephrase it as many times as necessary for the patient to understand. Do not ask sequential questions, such as, "Have you had nausea, vomiting, and diarrhea?" Break it into several questions. One of the concerns may be overlooked or included incorrectly.
- Give patients time to form an answer; some patients mentally translate English into their own language, decide on the response in their language, mentally translate it back into English, then relay it to you in English. Obviously, this is not as simple as processing all of the information in one language.
- Avoid slang; it is not appropriate in any exchange and does not translate well to other languages. Remember, too, that idioms are hard to translate.
- Be sure you completely understand the patient's response. Ask for clarification if you are not sure.
- Have consents, authorizations, billing forms, brochures, patient education, and so on, printed in the other languages common to your area. Post instructions in restrooms and reception areas in these languages also.
- To help establish rapport, learn several phrases in other languages. "Please," "Thank you," "Good day," and other greetings and pleasantries are easy to learn. Patients will appreciate your efforts to communicate and will be more responsive in return.

Remember that communication tactics vary with cultures. Some cultures require or reject close proxemics, others reject or expect eye contact. Patients who speak English as a second language will need communication adapted for their special needs.

IMPAIRMENT BARRIERS

Communication requires many sensory and receptive mental interactions to be effective. An impairment in any of the systems involved in communication interrupts the flow and leads to misunderstanding and frustration. In some of the instances listed below, a caregiver must be included to ensure that health care directives are followed or that you have a full and understandable history. In other situations, simply adjusting normal communication skills to accommodate an impairment allows the patient to participate in personal health care, which always should be the goal of patient interaction.

Hearing

Since many hearing losses are gradual, patients may not be aware they are missing or misunderstanding parts of the conversation, and may wonder why *you* have trouble communicating. Many patients refuse to admit they do not hear well, and trying to convince them may be more frustrating than productive. Adjust your communication to work with them until they realize they need corrective help.

Patients who demonstrate any of the following may have a hearing impairment:

- Flat speech patterns with little **inflection**, or variation in tone. We alter and vary our speech as we hear it, raising and lowering our pitch and tone for emphasis. Hearing-impaired patients may not change their speaking tones.
- Slurred or incomplete words. Patients may not be aware that they have not finished words or that the sounds were not distinct.
- Frequent requests that you repeat a statement. Questioning looks or puzzled expressions after you have spoken should tell you the patient did not understand.
- Apparent indifference to what you are saying. The patient may not know that you are speaking; we do not miss what we do not hear.
- A tendency to dominate the conversation. Patients may not be aware when you are speaking.

In any of these instances, suspect that patients have a hearing impairment and keep trying to communicate until you are sure they understand you (Box 2-3).

Hearing-impaired patients can read your cues and may be able to read your lips, but neither is fully effective. The following suggestions will help ensure your patient follows the conversation:

- Before beginning the conversation, alert the patient to the topic. For example, you may touch her and say, "Mrs. Smith, this is how you should change your dressing." She will know she must listen and will have an idea of the topic and the direction of the discussion.
- Position yourself directly in front of the patient with your face lighted for her convenience. She should be able to see you clearly to read all of your cues.
- Never turn away from the patient. Without a clear view of your face, and with your speech directed away, the patient is at a disadvantage.
- Speak clearly and distinctly, but do not exaggerate your facial movements. If your patient relies on reading lips, distorting your face and mouth makes it very hard to distinguish the words.
- Speak with moderate force, but lower your normal speaking pitch. Many patients lose higher tones first, but still can hear low-pitched tones. Shouting usually does not help and may distort what you are saying.
- As with other communication barriers, short words in short sentences are easier to interpret than complex words in lengthy sentences. The Rule of Fives works well for many barriers.

Box **2-3** **Hearing Impairments**

There are three main types of hearing impairment with degrees of loss within each:
- Conductive: This **impedance**, or barrier, is in the outer or middle ear and may be as simple as hardened cerumen (ear wax). It also may be otosclerosis (hardening of the structures of the ear), which interferes with the transmission of sound through the structures of the ear to the otic nerve. This type of hearing loss is correctable in most cases and responds well to clearing the ear canal with a simple cerumen impaction removal procedure, using a hearing aid, or replacing the stapes (a small bone in the middle ear involved in otosclerosis).
- Sensorineural: This deafness involves the otic nerve and sound transmission to the auditory (hearing) centers of the brain. It is a nerve impairment, rather than an impedance. At this time, if the loss is profound, the best solution is a device called a cochlear implant that transmits sound past the otic nerve to the brain. Traditional hearing aids may not work with this type of loss. Newer aids increase clarity (the quality of sound), without increasing volume. Simply increasing sound volume has a tendency to distort sounds for these patients.
- Mixed deafness: This is harder to diagnose and treat and may be a combination of both types of hearing loss. It is common in older patients and is then called **presbycusis** (literally "old hearing"). Since part of the problem is sensorineural, the solution may be difficult to determine. Hearing aids may not help, and raising your voice may make it worse.

Hearing losses range from very slight, with the patient losing only a few sounds such as "s" or "th," to profound, with a total loss of hearing, called **anacusis**.

- Keep distractions to a minimum to cut down on confusion and to make your words easier to understand.
- If you must cover your mouth for treatment purposes, as in masking, write what the patient needs to know or have someone at the patient's side to interpret.
- If the patient cannot understand you, use magic slates, chalkboards or note pads for writing. Pantomime and demonstration may help also.
- Learn as much sign language as you can, for your convenience and to show patients that you care. Patients will appreciate your efforts to communicate in their language.

Vision

Vision impairments range from hyperopia (farsightedness) and myopia (nearsightedness) to complete loss of vision. Vision-impaired patients can hear what you say but miss the cues and nonverbal language that help in an effective exchange. Patients cannot see you smiling, for example, though they may be perceptive and pick this up in your general tone of voice. In many cases, vision-impaired people develop other communication skills, such as more focused hearing and greater concentration. The following suggestions will help you interact with the vision-impaired patient.

- Reintroduce yourself each time you greet vision-impaired patients. Though your voice may be distinctive, it is embarrassing if you presume they remember you and they do not.
- Escort patients by having them take your arm, rather than taking theirs. This is more comfortable for patients and gives them a feeling of control.

- When you orient vision-impaired patients to an area, have them touch each item, such as the table or bed, counter or bedside table, chair, or room door. Scan the room for unsafe obstacles, such as trash containers or the physician's rolling stool. Be very aware of patients' safety.
- Knock each time you enter the room and let patients know who you are. Tell them when you must leave the room. Never leave patients alone without telling them that you are leaving.
- Explain each procedure and let patients know when you need to touch them. Remember that they cannot see that you have a thermometer in your hand or that you need to wrap the blood pressure cuff.
- Describe the sounds heard at each step of any procedure, such as those made by a whirring or clicking machine. Talk to patients about the steps of each procedure so that they know what you and the physician are doing and will know what to expect next.
- Recognize that raising your voice will not increase understanding. If the patient is also hearing impaired, follow the suggestions for communicating with hearing-impaired patients in addition to those listed here.
- If the patient is accompanied by a guide dog, be aware that the dog usually is allowed to go wherever the patient goes. Neither the patient nor the dog is comfortable if separated. These dogs are specially trained and are very good natured, but their primary interest is their owner. Do not distract the dog and do not handle or pet him unless the patient gives you permission.

Language

Patients lose the ability to speak or to understand speech for many reasons. As with other impairments, difficulty communicating by language ranges through degrees, such as the loss of a few words (dysphasia) to a total inability to speak (aphasia). Reasons for language impairments include a cerebrovascular accident, paralysis of the muscles used for speech, tracheostomy, laryngectomy, or impaired nervous system function.

The speech centers of the brain are contained in part of the left hemisphere (half of the brain) and in the frontal lobe near the areas that control the organs of speech (e.g., mouth, tongue, larynx). Oral communication requires that we choose the proper words from our memory banks and process them through functioning organs related to speech (e.g., tongue, larynx). When we respond, we must understand what we heard and form and transmit the words needed for a reply. All of this must be compared with nonverbal cues to fully interpret the message. Because this process is so complex, a breakdown or defect anywhere along the line disrupts communication (Box 2-4).

If patients have trouble speaking or responding to you, try these suggestions:

- Talk to patients in a calm, private place with few distractions. Processing information takes longer for these patients and will be more difficult if you or the patient cannot concentrate.
- Allow extra time for patients to understand what you are saying and to form responses.
- Treat patients with respect; do not treat them as you would a child. In many cases, intelligence is still intact.
- Use a normal tone of voice. Unless you suspect that patients are also hard of hearing, raising your voice will not help.
- Ask patients if they understand. You may be able to determine whether or not they comprehend just by the look in their eyes, even if they cannot answer "yes" or "no."
- Use short, simple phrases and words: the Rule of Fives. If the patient has any ability to speak, ask questions that require short answers.

Box **2-4** **Language Impairments**

Since so many sensory components are involved in communicating through language, there are many opportunities for impairments that interfere with getting our point across. These include an inability to write, to form speech, or to interpret visual symbols and visual cues. Several of the more common types include the following:

- Nonfluent or expressive: Although words may be formed, and communication may be possible, patients have trouble finding the right words. This is also called dysphasia, the term for difficulty forming speech. These patients cannot plan and organize normal speech. The brain knows what it wants to say but has forgotten where the words are stored. If the patient's intelligence is still intact, this is very frustrating. He may say, "I need my red tricycle," when he needs his medication, and may be angry when you do not understand what he thought he said. You will need great tact and diplomacy to help patients deal with frustration.

- Fluent or receptive: Patients may speak fairly well but they cannot process what they hear. Although hearing is usually intact and they can hear what you say, they cannot understand the words. Also, since we listen to ourselves as we speak to decide whether or not what we said was logical, fluent aphasics are not aware that what they said made no sense. These patients usually do not recognize that what they say tends to be garbled to the listener and usually see this as your problem, not theirs.

- Conductive: The brain can find and form the words, but the motor functions that tell our body what to do cannot transmit the impulses to the tongue, the throat, the larynx, or in some cases to any of the areas involved in speech. The words can be formed in the mind but cannot be spoken.

- Sensory: Patients cannot understand the spoken word if the auditory, or hearing, centers are involved, or the written word or symbols if the visual centers are involved. If both are affected, patients cannot understand either spoken or written communication. We can compensate for a loss of one sensory factor by applying the guidelines for communicating with hearing- or vision-impaired patients. If both are affected, communication will be very difficult.

- Global: This patient has lost the ability to express and to receive any form of communication. If his intelligence is still intact, the frustration is devastating; he can neither understand you nor help you understand him.

- Certain types of language impairments also affect the writing areas of the brain. If this is true for this patient, use pictures or flash cards and have the patient point to those that are appropriate.
- Give positive feedback to encourage patients to continue to try.

Expect patients to be very frustrated when they cannot communicate. In many instances, they know exactly what they want to say and cannot form the words. This increases anger; be patient and do not take the anger personally. Remember, the patient is frustrated with the situation, not with you.

An interesting aspect of language impairment involves singing. Singing is not processed in the same area of the brain as spoken language. Patients with some types of language impairment may not be able to form words properly or find the needed words but may have no problem singing what they want to say.

Much of our socialization and survival involves our ability to communicate; never stop trying to communicate with persons who cannot respond. Always talk to these patients and explain everything just as you would to patients who respond verbally. Listening to and processing words is a part of speech formation and may help the patient learn to speak again.

Cognitive

The ability to think through information and to respond appropriately is so complex that disabilities that disrupt thought processes also hinder communication. These include brain injuries as a result of trauma or disease (such as a cerebrovascular accident), degenerative changes (such as senile dementia or Alzheimer's disease), mental retardation, and many other causes. Although hearing and sight may be intact, patients cannot organize their thoughts to understand you and cannot help you understand them in return.

Severely cognitively impaired patients usually are accompanied by a caregiver to whom you will direct most of your interview or instruction; however, do not exclude the patient. As with any other impairment or challenge, patients need to feel as involved as possible and may make small, limited decisions. Since disabilities vary so widely, some level of interaction may be possible. Interacting with others helps keep patients in touch with reality and with their environment.

The following suggestions work in many situations involving cognitively impaired patients.

- Consult with caregivers as you communicate with patients. They live with these barriers every day and have developed ways to communicate effectively.
- Interact in an environment as free of distractions as possible. Cognitively impaired persons are easily distracted and find it hard to concentrate in a noisy, busy area.
- Assume the patient will not remember you or your instructions from your last interaction. Approach these patients as if the situation is new each time.
- Look directly at the patient and engage his attention before beginning. Touching the patient may bring his attention to you. Holding his hand and talking directly to him may help keep his attention focused on you and your words.
- Lower the pitch of your voice and do not talk in a sing-song, child-like voice. Patients may pay more attention if you speak in soft, low-pitched tones. Never shout; they may be easily frightened.
- Use the Rule of Fives. Use easy concepts in short, easy sentences. Pictures and drawings are also appropriate.
- Give small, limited choices, such as, "Would you rather I take your temperature first, or weigh you first?" Small choices give patients a degree of control and increase self-esteem.
- Closed-ended questions are appropriate in this situation. Open-ended questions may be confusing. (See Chapter 3, "Gathering Information," for more discussion of these types of questions.)
- Never correct patients and never argue. It does not matter whether they are right or wrong. Trying to convince the cognitively impaired patient is frustrating for both of you. Agree and continue with your tasks.
- Praise the patient for cooperation. Respond positively to efforts to contribute.

Medical Illness

Many patients who are not particularly ill are in our presence for health maintenance, recovery from an injury, or check-ups following acute illness. Patients who are not coping with symptoms of illness have one less barrier to overcome. However, most of our patients are acutely, chronically, or profoundly ill when they need our attention. This can be one of our most difficult challenges.

Patients who are actively sick cannot listen to anything other than what is happening within the body. Pain, nausea, vertigo, and other symptoms of illness make it hard to communicate beyond the most basic information needed to relieve the most disturbing concerns. Even patients who are not acutely or actively ill have trouble concentrating because of the psychological noise whirling around in their brains. Worrisome thoughts fill their minds, such as, "How will this affect my career, my marriage, my life?" "How can I pay for this?" "Will I be scarred, crippled, sick for the rest of my life?" "Will I die from this?" Nothing that you say at this time is as important as what is shouting over your voice. Trying to communicate about topics other than relief at this time will increase stress and may make the situation worse for the patient.

If at all possible, relieve as many of the overwhelming problems as possible. After alerting the physician for orders and caring for the acute symptoms, allow time for relief measures to calm the patient before continuing. Keep the interaction as brief as possible at this time with only the information immediately necessary. The following suggestions may help.

- Read the patient's cues regarding relief of symptoms, such as a returning awareness and an increase in attention to you and the surroundings. Trying to communicate when symptoms are overwhelming is frustrating for both of you.
- Touch the patient and gain her attention to return her awareness to you so that she will concentrate on what you must say.
- Keep communication as simple as possible; limit topics to "need-to-know-now." More extensive information can be exchanged later.

When symptoms are manageable again, follow other communication guidelines you feel will help with this patient.

THE STRESSED PATIENT

Even patients who present for nothing more serious than a recheck or routine physical examination build stress as they wait, wondering if the twinge of pain they felt 2 weeks ago meant something after all. Instructing patients who are stressed is covered in Chapter 4, "Educating Patients," and Chapter 5, "Communicating Wellness," covers how stress affects the body. At this point, we are most concerned with ways to relieve the stress naturally felt by patients as they work through the often frightening medical environment.

It is very difficult to communicate with patients overwhelmed by stress. Patients who are very ill are under great stress, of course, and even those who are mildly or acutely ill are burdened by the possibility of illness. Our role in communicating with these patients is to calm and soothe and to recognize that stress is a side effect of illness, much like a fever or a rash. In many cases, as we will see, stress is itself the cause of illness. Before we can accurately measure vital signs and record our observations regarding the patient's current state, we must respond to the racing heart and high blood pressure by attempting to relieve stress.

As with many of our barriers, a calm, relaxing environment relieves much of the patient's tension. Trying to communicate in an area with many distractions and high tension is not productive. If you recognize that your patient is under great stress, the following suggestions may help relieve the situation before it **escalates**, or increases, into something more serious.

- Acknowledge to yourself and to the patient that she has a right to feel stressed. The medical environment can be frightening, with its foreign language and strange, invasive procedures.
- Speak calmly and spend time just chatting about the patient's family, job, and so on, while you progress through the early portions of the interaction. You may uncover clues to stress from his personal or professional life, which may be the primary problem.
- Lower the pitch of your voice and slow your speech patterns to soothe the patient's anxiety.
- As with any exchange, sitting across from the patient, eye-to-eye, in a relaxed but professional manner inspires confidence and communicates compassion, both of which are calming.
- Allow the patient as many choices as possible to reinforce a sense of control. If she feels she has choices, one of her choices may be to approach the situation more calmly. If the situation is very stressful, as in a dreaded diagnosis, you may have to help the patient make decisions about health care. She may not be able to decide anything at this time.
- If the patient becomes too stressed to cooperate, call for help from the physician.

THE ANGRY, HOSTILE, OR COMBATIVE PATIENT

If you cannot relieve the patient's stress, the situation may deteriorate into a full anxiety attack or may result in a patient who is unable to control emotional outbursts. Some patients use **belligerence,** or angry stubbornness, to hide from their fear as they tell themselves, "I'm not afraid, I'm mad!"

These patients generally are not angry with their health care providers, unless there is reason to be because of some problem caused by the health care worker. Anger is usually a reaction to loss of control. Patients may become hostile and progress to either verbal abuse or, less frequently, physical abuse in the form of combativeness. Since you are more approachable and safer than the physician, the anger may be directed at you.

If you find yourself in this upsetting situation, the following suggestions may help:

- Do not take the anger personally. Respect the patient's feelings and the need to relieve stress by venting. Anger and loss of control are symptoms of illness; think of them as you would a fever.
- Give calm, soft answers and responses. Listen intently with attentive body language and observe body cues closely for either a decrease or increase in the patient's anger.
- Determine whether the feelings are valid. If the anger has a basis in fact, and you or your agency is at fault, try to make amends. Explain how you will make every effort to correct the problem. Do not admit guilt or fault, and do not blame anyone else; simply do what you can to correct the situation and talk through the problem.
- Never argue in return. This absolutely will increase distress and anger.
- Gently set limits for what you will not tolerate, such as profanity or verbal abuse.
- Call for the physician if you cannot calm the patient.
- Document the entire incident: the source of the anger, how the patient expressed it, and your actions to correct the situation.

If the situation deteriorates further and the patient becomes aggressive and combative, use great caution as you follow these suggestions.

- Do not let the patient come between you and the door. Always have a clear path to an escape route.
- Move slowly and in full view to avoid any perceived threat to the patient.

- Again, but with caution, set limits and tell the patient that these actions are unacceptable.
- Call for help from coworkers and the physician. If the situation is openly dangerous, someone must call 911 and summon help.
- When the crisis is over, document all that happened and how it was handled.
- Learn from the situation and be aware of verbal and nonverbal cues that might lead to other confrontations.

AGE BARRIERS

Any age different than our own is a potential barrier to effective communication. Obviously, we would not interact with a very young child or with someone very much older in the same way we would with someone our own age. For example, it is harder to give care to young children who cannot communicate with us and who do not understand why we must do the things we do. We may have trouble communicating with older adults with degenerative illnesses and sensory impairments. If we can remember how our levels of maturity and perception have changed through the years, it will be easier to interact with different age groups by understanding their changing characteristics.

Children

Caring for children with levels of development from newborn to preteen is particularly challenging. There are several theories of growth and development, but one of the more prominent models was developed by the Swiss psychologist Jean Piaget (1896-1980) when he divided the levels of ability to think and reason along the following lines.
- Sensorimotor activities from birth to age 2: Children develop and progress during this time through primitive reflexes to more complex thought patterns, such as the following:
  - Sucking and rooting (the ability to bring things to the mouth)
  - Eye/hand (seeing an object and reaching for it)
  - Discovering self-rewarding activities (thumb-sucking, playing with a favorite object)
  - Anticipating ("I see the bottle. It must be for me.")
  - Exploring ("If I pull this lamp cord, I wonder what will happen.")
  - Verbal skills also develop during this stage as children learn to communicate and interact with caregivers.
- Preoperational thought from 2 to 7: This age is self-centered; these children believe the world revolves around them. They can determine quantities ("He has more jelly beans than I do.") and size ("See how big I am."), and are mastering their environment ("Kindergarten was fun, but big school is scary." "If Mom won't let me do it, maybe Dad will."). They begin to learn from friends in their playgroup and at school and feel the need to blend with their peers.
- Concrete thought from 7 to 11: With greater reasoning skills, this age understands that things and people change, that you might have a point of view different from theirs, and they can consider and accept differences of opinion. They understand abstract concepts and are beginning to exercise self-determination, called **autonomy**. Peer groups frequently are more influential than family at this age.
- Formal operational thought from 11 to 15: With deepening and developing levels of the social skills listed above, this age group recognizes its unique personality and begins to question authority for the full autonomy needed for adulthood.

All of these stages of development and comprehension require different approaches to communication. Understanding the patient's ability to comprehend before you begin makes interaction easier for everyone. Never expect a child or young person to understand or react on a level beyond the current life stage. For example, a 5-year-old child is not capable of the same level of reasoning we expect of a 9-year-old, but we should expect the 5-year-old to react at a higher level of development than a 3-year-old.

When a child is ill at any age, developmental stages can regress. Young children who are potty-trained and have given up the bottle may take a step back to an earlier dependence. A 7-year-old who normally would not want to cuddle on her mother's lap may need the reassurance of being held by her during a procedure. This is particularly hard for the preteen who wants desperately to be grown-up but still needs to be comforted during illness.

Young children frequently see illness and treatment procedures as punishment. They cannot understand why they feel so bad and why we have to hurt them to make them feel better. They may be very angry, combative, and, at least for this time, truly hard to love. Accept this behavior as a life stage and a symptom of illness. Children in the early ages are no more to blame for this reaction than for a rash or fever in response to illness.

To interact effectively, keep the environment bright, colorful, child-friendly, and safe. Being ill is not fun, but it does not have to be frightening. These suggestions may help:

- Be aware that looking up at a large adult is scary. For better rapport, position yourself eye-to-eye with the child. Raise the child to your level or lower yourself to the child's level.
- Pitch your voice low and gentle. Loud, forced, or funny voices may be frightening rather than calming.
- Never surprise children by touching them without warning. Move slowly and calmly, and let them see what you are doing. The only exception to this suggestion is an injection. Warn children before injections, but they may become more frightened if they actually see the syringe.
- Let them ask questions, and answer at an age-appropriate level. Keep trying to provide answers until the child understands and has no further questions. If you think the questions are a delaying tactic, take appropriate steps to continue with treatment.
- Listen as attentively to children as you do to adults. They sense when you care and when you do not.
- Play for a few moments before you begin working with children and, if reasonable, let them handle equipment. Children may even pretend to assist you by holding a piece of equipment as you place your hand over theirs and work through the procedural steps.
- Never scold children for crying and resisting when they are stressed or frightened, as this is normal behavior. If the child is old enough to reason, explaining why the procedure is needed may be all you need to help the situation.
- Let parents hold children as much as possible for treatment or procedures. This is comforting to both parent and child.
- As with adults, stress in a child's world may bring on phantom illnesses. For instance, the tummyache this morning may be a very real response to the stress of a situation at school and should be investigated by parents if there is no organic reason for the symptom.
- Reward children with stickers and praise for good behavior, but do not belittle them if their fear was greater than their need to cooperate.
- Be very careful using idioms and other expressions with small children. Children have vivid imaginations and can become confused and frightened by things they hear. For example, if the child hears you say, "She will need a CAT scan," she may be understandably upset (Fig. 2-2).

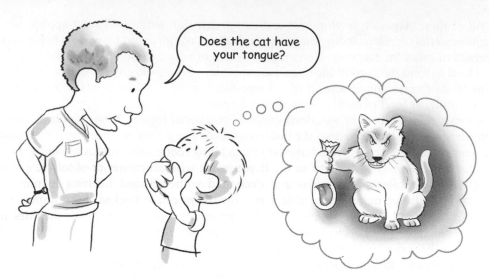

Figure 2-2

Chronically ill children who have spent much of their young lives in hospitals are likely to fear abandonment; however, much of their anxiety can be relieved if you allow parents or caregivers to be an active part of medical care. These children usually become prematurely receptive to cues, always wondering, "Will this person hurt me?" They may be unusually resistant or equally unusually passive. Children who have given up trying to control the pain of medical procedures sometimes do not even cry when most children would scream with fear or anger. Healthy resistance is actually more natural than passive acceptance. Handle all children with care and respect, but be especially receptive to the needs of chronically ill children.

Families coping with sick children are in crisis, particularly if the child is chronically ill. Parents and caregivers are usually physically, emotionally, and financially exhausted. Parents may be in different stages of grief (see Chapter 6, "Communicating Through the Grief Process") and cannot offer each other much-needed emotional support. Siblings frequently act out their anger and jealousy and may present with phantom illnesses to try to direct much-needed attention to themselves. Unrelieved tension and stress may lead to anger all around—the children cannot express their feelings and the parents suppress theirs. Unfortunately, many families with a seriously ill child do not survive the situation intact. They need your support and understanding through this difficult time.

Teenagers

Teenagers present such challenges that a new division of medicine was developed for their specific needs. Adolescent medicine is directed at the young person who is not quite a child but not yet an adult. These are usually years of good health, but it is also a time of great experimentation and high-risk behavior for many young people. Various statistics show that more than half have had unprotected sex by their late teens, sexually transmitted diseases are on the rise in this age group, they have notoriously poor nutrition, and many are already set in a sedentary lifestyle. Many are sexually mature but without the psychological and physical maturity to cope with the consequences. Clearly, this group needs an approach different than young children or responsible adults.

Many young people who are not quite ready for adult medicine understandably do not want to be considered pediatric patients. Medical facilities that include pediatric patients usually are stocked with magazines directed toward young children or their parents and are filled with baby toys. These young people are reaching for maturity and independence and now find themselves back in a child-like atmosphere. They usually are resentful enough at being ill and relying on parents again without being reminded that they are not as far out of childhood as they would like to be. If you work with a number of older children, an area set aside from crying babies and decorated with teenaged interests in mind will make this age group more comfortable. Teen-only rooms can be stocked with computers and video games, and with age-appropriate posters and magazines. Inpatient facilities may have a room away from the treatment areas to separate patients from the constant reminders of illness.

Teenagers can be very self-centered, self-critical, and insecure; some see every problem as a unique disaster. Even a pimple is forever. While they are trying to be mature, an illness pulls them back into a reluctant dependent stage. Just as they enter an autonomous, authority-defying stage, authorities are telling them what to do again. Expect resistance; this is natural. The following suggestions, and a high measure of patience, understanding, and good humor help the interaction:

- Talk with the young person alone if possible. Many young people cannot open up to their parents, partly because of the need to loosen bonds, and partly because not all families are as functional as we would like. Ask in private whether teens would like a parent to be part of the procedure or examination. If the teen asks that parents not attend, the issue is private. The Legal Eagle box covers confidentiality issues for the teenaged patient.
- Although teen patients may presume to know everything, assume that they do not and proceed with caution to explain what you must do. Listen more than you talk. You may learn by words or cues what you need to know and what they do not understand.
- Let teens make as many decisions as possible. They need to feel in control and will be more cooperative if their personal feelings are included in decisions involving their care.

 ## LEGAL EAGLE

Various state and federal regulations mandate patient confidentiality, even when communicating with a parent about a minor child. Most states have laws that prevent health care workers from speaking to parents about their child's sexual history, drug use, sexually transmitted diseases, or pregnancies. Parents often become upset about these regulations, especially since their health insurance may still be required to pay for the services. You need to know your state's laws and follow the policy of your work place. In certain situations, minor children may sign a HIPAA release form and allow parents access to their health care records and treatments.

- Teens distrust authority and resent and resist an authoritative attitude on your part. However, you need to limit immature behavior and set limits for what you will and will not accept.
- Give teens privacy. They are at a very self-conscious age and will resent it if you intrude on personal space.
- Be alert for reports of fatigue. This may be a sign of infectious mononucleosis, drug behavior, or depression. Reports of poor schoolwork or disinterest in social activities should also be documented.
- Use every opportunity to educate teens regarding high-risk behavior. This age does not see the dangers in drugs, alcohol, sex, and other high-risk activities. Teens may resist your attempts, but some of the information may register.
- Adjust patient education for teen interests. Posters and brochures featuring teen idols with appropriate messages are more effective than the same literature created for older patients.
- Know that this age group is very aware of an insincere or judgmental attitude. They are more perceptive than young children, who have not yet learned to identify attitudes, or older adults, who are preoccupied by other stressors. Teenaged patients will close you out immediately if they sense you are not sincere or are judging them by your own standards.

Adults

The adult years are generally years of good health devoted to establishing families and careers. Most adult patients present for health maintenance or for an occasional acute illness or traumatic injury. Some, of course, develop serious illnesses, but most enjoy many years of productive emotional, social, and professional growth.

This is also the time of the "sandwich" generation, caught between growing children and aging parents. The stress of coping may be overwhelming and may lead to many vague symptoms with few significant findings to support a diagnosis. These may include stress-related headaches, shoulder and back pain from tension, or gastrointestinal complaints related to diet or stress. Frequently, there are no organic reasons for the complaints, but patients still need relief from the symptoms. Unfortunately, finding and addressing the cause of these concerns can be very difficult.

Since these adults are frequently about the same age and in the same situations as many health care workers, communication is usually fairly easy. These suggestions should enhance the interaction:

- Know as much as you can about the patient. How stressful is his job? Has the job recently been terminated? How many roles is she juggling? How does she respond to crises? What are his social habits, such as drinking and smoking? All of these factors affect health and should be discussed during most interactions.
- Without lecturing, and with sincere compassion, offer preventive patient education to ensure good health habits. Make the interaction and education as specific as possible so that patients feel the information was personally designed for their problems.
- Remind patients of the need for **respite**, or relief, from their many roles and remind them that they need strong social support groups.

- Allow patients time to talk about their stress. Talking it through may be the most therapeutic response during these stress-filled years.

The Older Adult

Our older populations are growing as many people live longer, healthier lives. However, we are still responsible for the care of the degenerative and chronic disorders that add to the adjustments this age group must make. Reactions to aging differ considerably depending on the patient's financial, physical, emotional, and social resources. Patients confined in a facility where someone else makes all decisions and where there are few opportunities for self-expression feel differently than older adults who still live independently with physical and financial freedom to come and go at will. Older adults in good physical health with adequate social and financial support can remain vital and active for many years.

We retain our central personality as we mature. Grouchy young people usually become even grouchier as they age. Those who see life as a challenging adventure will anticipate each stage of maturity with pleasure. Those who have nothing to look forward to except the next meal and directed arts and crafts, or who are insecure about health and finances, become understandably depressed. This is a time when many older adults engage in "life-review," remembering earlier, happier years. If you have time, listen to their stories; you may be fascinated, you may learn, and your lonely, older patient will love having an audience.

Most of the older patients in your care retain all of the skills expected of patients of any age; however, advanced age may bring about many of the communication barriers discussed previously. These suggestions may help in either situation:

- Never treat older patients as if they were children. This is referred to as infantilizing and is insulting to the patient.
- Always use the patient's surname and title, such as Mr. Smith or Mrs. Jones, unless expressed permission is given for first names. As a matter of respect, it still is not a good idea to place the relationship on such a personal basis.
- Since many systems, such as vision and hearing, are less acute, allow more time for care and procedures.
- Check the lighting and safety of the facility's rooms from an older person's perspective. Dim lights and clutter are dangerous when vision and mobility are limited.
- Make sure patients understand instructions and help by making suggestions that compensate for memory lapses, such as medication dispensers and calendars with treatment instructions.
- Respect the needs of older adults to remain independent but include caregivers whenever appropriate.
- If patients must return frequently for treatment, set appointments for each visit for the same day and time at the patient's convenience. This makes it easier for them to remember.
- Help with home safety suggestions by offering patient education material that covers ways to compensate for losses in sight, hearing, and balance.

People of all ages sense whether you sincerely care about their welfare and will respond to a compassionate, professional approach. Patients of all ages are concerned with how illness will affect who they are at each life stage. The first step in a return to health is establishing an effective relationship between the patient and the health care environment; this is one of your greatest responsibilities (see the Spotlight on Success box).

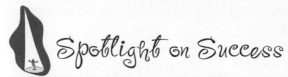

Spotlight on Success

While you are helping an elderly female patient dress, the patient states, "With my arthritis, I can't even tie my own shoes anymore. Getting old is not fun." How should you respond? It is very important not to belittle the person making the statement or take this concern lightly. For example, do not say, "It's no big deal. I'll tie your shoes for you." Or "Just get shoes with Velcro®." Instead, use this opportunity to explore the patient's ability to care for herself and how she feels about her limitations. A good opening statement might be, "What other things do you find hard to do?" After gathering additional information, speak with the physician. This patient may benefit from working with an occupational therapist. You can make a difference in someone's life by taking the time to communicate and explore the hidden messages that patients send to you.

PERSONAL BIASES

Perhaps the most difficult barrier to overcome is also the least obvious. We are immediately aware of many barriers, such as age, physical disabilities, and language, but we may be unaware that closely held personal beliefs can interfere with communication as effectively as any of the more obvious obstacles we have discussed. Since these **biases** frequently are based on cultural differences, review the suggestions for overcoming culture-based barriers.

Stereotyping and Prejudice

Stereotyping gathers together in our mind an entire group of people who are different from the group to which we belong. We tend to see our group as a diverse blend of independent personalities; we may see other groups as all the same, molded into sameness rather than as individuals. This means that stereotyping disregards individual self-worth and the personal differences that make us distinctly who we are. We generally assume that the group to which we belong has superior qualities, which helps us maintain group self-esteem and keeps our group together. In an effort to make ourselves feel better about our group, we may see others as somewhat inferior, making us feel better at someone else's expense. For example, though we may think highly of those with more money or education, we still have not allowed individuals to register as separate from the group. This in turn diminishes their self-worth, making us feel superior by being distinctly individual.

Carried to the next level, stereotyping leads to prejudice. In this bias, we prejudge everyone by our ideas regarding the stereotyped group to which he belongs. We may be prejudiced for or against a certain group, although the term usually is used negatively. For instance, we may be more accepting of a certain type of patient than we are others. In that case, we are prejudiced for one group and against the other. This leads to preferential treatment for certain patients, as covered previously in "Other Cultural Barriers," in this chapter.

If we have a strongly developed personality with adequate self-esteem, we do not need prejudice to feel good about ourselves. We will not need to see someone else as inferior to recognize our own self-worth. If you find you do not like a patient, and realize that this is based on prejudice, analyze why the relationship is difficult. Are you uncomfortable with the differences? Are your beliefs about yourself and your group threatened? Can you understand what it is about this patient that bothers you? Understanding why you do not like certain types of patients helps you grow as an effective communicator and is vital to overcoming unacceptable, unprofessional behavior. Biases lead to negative treatment, such as avoiding patients, rushed treatment, and superficial interaction. This in turn leads to poor communication and ineffective patient relationships. Without strong efforts at understanding, stereotyping leads to prejudice, and prejudice leads to **discrimination**.

We can overcome prejudice by working with varied groups of people with all participants on an equal basis. If one group takes a superior or supervisory position, prejudice will continue. Working toward a common goal for a good purpose, such as in a health care setting or charitable situation, makes all participants feel good about themselves and breaks down the barriers of prejudice.

Although it is difficult to treat all patients equally well, or even to like each one, many of the stereotypical and prejudiced reactions that we see in health care interfere with our ability to give objective and compassionate health care. It is our responsibility to work toward overcoming every barrier that blocks effective communication.

 ## Taking the Chapter to Work

Now, let's meet Elisa and Gwen and see how they have applied this chapter information in the workplace.

Elisa is working in an endocrinology clinic. Elisa starts every morning by organizing her patient charts. She notices that Mr. Ollie is scheduled for an appointment at 10 a.m. for insulin administration education. According to the receptionist, the patient is having trouble seeing the numbers on the syringe. Elisa looks in the chart and notices that Mr. Ollie has cataracts and retinopathy. She knows that retinopathy is a common eye disorder that affects diabetic patients and makes visualizing small items difficult. So, Elisa finds the educational tools available for diabetic patients and obtains an insulin syringe magnifying glass. She also prints copies of insulin administration sheets in large print. Elisa puts these items with Mr. Ollie's chart. When Mr. Ollie arrives for his appointment, the education session is completed in an organized and prompt manner because all of the needed materials were ready with the chart.

Gwen is working in a pediatrician's office. She is caring for a 9-year-old boy who needs to have blood drawn. Gwen knows that this age group has concrete thought processes and thrives on autonomy. Using this knowledge, she plans her communication dialogue to include greater reasoning statements than she would have if the patient had been 5 years old. Gwen successfully draws the blood without a problem.

Beyond the Classroom Exercises

Your Assignment Board

The following exercises will help you use your new knowledge. Place a check beside the assignments your instructor has given you. When you have completed the assignment, place a check in the completed column.

		Assigned	*Completed*
Checking Your Comprehension	(Textbook)	❏	❏
Expanding Critical Thinking	(Textbook)	❏	❏
Communication Surfer Exercises	(Textbook and Internet)	❏	❏
Communication Tree Branch #2	(CD-ROM)	❏	❏
Voice Mail Message #2	(CD-ROM)	❏	❏

Checking Your Comprehension

Write a brief answer for each of the following assignments.
1. List three barriers that could affect your ability to form a therapeutic relationship with a patient.
2. Explain the difference between a matriarchal and a patriarchal society.
3. List five methods that you can use to communicate effectively with a patient who does not speak English.
4. Define three types of hearing loss and give three examples on how you can communicate effectively with a patient who has each type.
5. Explain how a visual impairment can affect someone's ability to communicate effectively.
6. How can a medical illness affect a patient's ability to communicate effectively?
7. How does stress affect a patient's ability to communicate effectively?
8. Explain the various developmental stages and how you can promote communication throughout each stage.

Expanding Critical Thinking

1. How might you react in these situations? Would your feelings affect your ability to communicate effectively?
   a. An elderly uncle brings a young female patient into a clinic. Would you see this as inappropriate? Could you accept the situation as culturally proper for the family's dominant male?
   b. Your patient's culture forbids physical mutilation but the patient needs surgery. Do you think the power of communication could make him change his mind?
   c. Your elderly patient holds tightly to an **amulet**, or charm, during a painful procedure, and asks if she may take it with her during surgery.
2. Name and describe the cultures represented in your area. Did you include cultures of wealth, age, profession, and education? Describe the communication challenges within each culture?
3. Think of the wealthy people you know; now think of the poor that you know. Describe how they are alike, how they differ from each other, and how they differ from you. Are there any differences in communicating with either group?
4. List 10 types of stereotyping remarks you have heard and may have used. Include remarks such as "Old people are sick and forgetful," and "Young people are so rude." How do these remarks, and those that you remember, diminish the groups involved?

 ## Communication Surfer Exercises

1. Using a search engine, type in the word *stress*. How many sites did you find? What word(s) can you use to narrow your search to find sites that would help you communicate effectively with a patient who is experiencing stress? Using the sites that you found, create a list of at least 15 ways to help a patient who is experiencing stress.

2. You are caring for a patient with a visual impairment. Find the three sites that offer information about local resources for visually impaired people. How could a visually impaired patient access the Internet? What resources could help this patient enjoy the benefits of using a computer and the Internet?

3. A 15-year old patient tells you that she enjoys chat rooms. How many different style chat rooms are on the Internet? Create a list of chats rooms that would be appropriate for this age group. What types of chat rooms would be inappropriate for this age group? How would you communicate this information to a teenager?

3

GATHERING INFORMATION: LEARNING ABOUT THE PATIENT

LEARNING OBJECTIVES

Upon successfully completing this chapter, you will be able to:

- Differentiate between open-ended questions and closed-ended questions and give examples of both.
- Contrast *reflecting* and *clarifying* and give examples of both.
- Explain the importance of clarifying in an interview.
- Give examples of leading the interview, and explain how this is different from asking leading questions.
- Explain why silences should be encouraged in an interview.
- Explain why summarizing information is important.
- Explain the difference between hearing and listening
- List ways to enhance active listening.

KEY TERMS

Acronym
Algorithm
Chief complaint
Clarify, clarifying

Gate, gating
Paraphrasing
Reflecting
Sequence

Sequential
Subjective
Summarizing

Test Your Communication IQ

Before reading this chapter, take this short self-assessment test. Decide which statements are true and which are false.

1. The policy and procedure manual can serve as a guide to make patient interviews complete and relevant.
2. It is important to review the patient's medical history before beginning an interaction.
3. Patient responses give you subjective information.
4. "Do you have nausea, vomiting, and diarrhea?" is an acceptable question to ask a patient with abdominal pain.
5. "You are taking your medicine, aren't you?" is a good question to determine patient compliance.
6. The chief complaint is always the main reason a patient seeks care.
7. Periods of silence may help a confused patient gather his thoughts.
8. Gating is an essential skill to develop when interviewing patients.

Results

Statements four, five, and six are false. All other statements are true. How did you do? Read the chapter to find out more about these topics.

GATHERING INFORMATION

One of the most puzzling concerns for students beginning clinical experience involves therapeutic interaction and determining patient needs. This leads to the question: "How will I know what to ask?" Unfortunately, there is no single best answer. The questions needed to determine the root of a patient's problem are as different as the presenting illnesses and the patients themselves. For example, presume you ask Mr. Martin, "How may we help you today?" and he answers, "I think I have the flu." This simple, very common response leads to a multitude of questions. The progression of questions is very different if Mr. Martin is young and otherwise healthy than if he is elderly with hypertension and insulin-dependent diabetes mellitus. Every question and every response will be as individual as each patient's history and current concern. A skilled professional learns to follow a logical progression from the simplest "What can we do for you?" or "How may I help you?" to the most probing, in-depth evaluation of the patient's problem.

To make gathering information easier, and to ensure that all necessary points are covered, some specialties develop **algorithms** for specific complaints (Fig. 3-1). An algorithm states an issue and offers paths to follow, depending on the patient's answer at each step. For example, if the answer to a specific question is "yes," a suggestion for the next question follows. If the answer is "no," the next question follows a different pattern. This works well in some instances but may not allow for individual responses. An algorithm system may be too focused for individual patients, or too general for a focused interview. However, even the most inadequate algorithm at least leads in a general direction of questioning that the physician prefers.

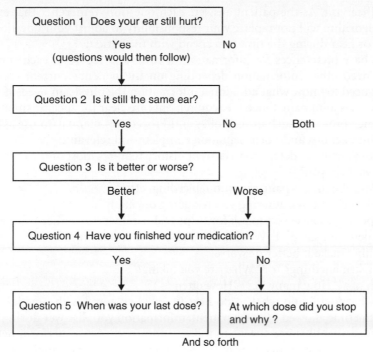

Figure 3-1
Example of an interviewing or questioning algorithm for a check-up visit after an ear infection.

Another tool to help with a preset plan, and to cover as much necessary information as possible, is the use of **acronyms**. An acronym is a simple phrase or word with a question coordinated for each letter. Acronyms are easy to remember. Questions may be either general or specific, with additional questions added based on each answer you receive. For example, Box 3-1 shows an acronym—MDVISIT—that could be used for a routine

Box **3-1**   **Acronym**

This is an example of a common acronym used for a general visit.

Medications—Are you taking prescribed medications or over-the-counter (OTC) preparations? Can you list them? How and when do you take each one? Do you need refills?

Diet—Describe your normal day's diet. How is your appetite? Have you lost or gained weight recently?

Visits—Have you visited another physician or been in the emergency department (ED) (or emergency room [ER]) since the last time we saw you?

Injuries—Have you had any injuries/falls/accidents recently? Describe what happened.

Symptoms—Are you experiencing any new problems/symptoms?

Information—Do you have questions regarding your medical care?

Treatments—How are you performing the treatments the doctor discussed on your last visit?

physician's office visit. As the patient answers each question, remember that even the best acronym or algorithm will not replace your responsibility to adjust your questions based on what you see or hear during the time you spend with the patient.

Physicians have preferences for information to cover and record at each encounter, and then usually need other information depending on the patient's current complaint. For example, you need to know what additional information the physician needs if the concern is chest pain versus joint pain. Once the requirements are clear for specific situations, record this in an agency protocol, such as the Policy and Procedures manual, to use as a guide and to help keep interactions and documentation complete and relevant.

Talking with patients to determine a current history requires most of the following points:
- "How may we help you?"
- "Can you describe the ....(pain, sensation, bleeding, etc.)?"
- "How long has this been bothering you (or going on, etc.)?"
- "What happened to cause you to ask for help? Did it get worse, bother you more, etc?"
- "Has it happened in the past? What did you do about it that time?"
- "Does anything make it better or worse?"
- "Have you taken anything?" or "What are you taking?"
- "How much ....?" "How many ....?" "How often ....?"

Knowing what to ask and what to do next is a skill acquired with practice. With rising demands on the time allowed for each patient, information you discover during the interaction or exchange should suggest steps to follow and procedures to perform before passing the patient's care to the next member of the health care team. For example, consider a situation involving an elderly patient (Mr. Martin) who has chronic health problems (insulin-dependent diabetes mellitus) along with an acute illness such as a virus (described above). In addition to routinely checking his vital signs, you should also check his blood sugar level and question him to make sure he is following his health care routine. Document this information and report to his physician. If the situation involves a younger, otherwise healthy patient, gather and record basic information, but glucose levels are not necessary. As another example, if Mrs. Smith complains of burning on urination, your responsibility and scope of practice might include obtaining a clean-catch midstream urine specimen in addition to routine vital signs. Gathering additional information by performing appropriate preliminary procedures expands on the current health complaint and provides the physician with information needed for a full diagnosis. Without full knowledge of the patient's past and current history, vital information may be overlooked, which may require backtracking and duplicated effort. If you do not follow a possible line of questioning and miss an issue of concern, time is wasted while the physician, instead of you, determines the full scope of the complaint. Our goal is to know as much as possible about our patients by gathering information effectively before any procedure begins.

SETTING THE STAGE

Current information is gathered and recorded with every patient contact, whether in person, by phone, or by written communication. Since most patient contact is on a personal basis, this text presumes that you and the patient are sharing a verbal exchange.

Whenever possible, the medical environment should be professional but friendly, not cold and sterile. Warm, bright colors and a comfortable setting help put patients at ease. The area should be private with no interruptions to threaten confidentiality or to disrupt the flow of

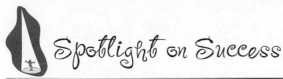

Spotlight on Success

You never get another chance to make a first impression, and, unfortunately, a bad first impression is hard to change. If you are neat, clean, and organized, patients and other health care providers are more likely to respect you and your professionalism. They will feel you are more knowledgeable than others who are disorganized and unprofessional. Patients feel more relaxed and communicate more freely with someone they feel is professional. Workers with these skills are more likely to be trusted with responsibility and to advance in their careers.

the conversation. Practice good personal hygiene and proper grooming to make a good impression and to establish or maintain rapport and respect for your professionalism (see the Spotlight on Success box).

The following suggestions should help make each exchange of information more effective:
- Before you begin, review the patient's chart. Knowing the patient's background and medical history shows that you are interested and concerned and gives you an idea of the questions you should ask.
- Sit in a comfortably relaxed and open position; crossed arms transmit rejection, rigid posture is intimidating, and slouching is unprofessional.
- Sit at the patient's level, face-to-face. If it is culturally acceptable to the patient, maintain eye contact.
- Show your interest by appropriate facial and nonverbal expressions, such as smiling and nodding.
- Listen attentively and stay centered on the conversation. Patients are aware when you are not listening.
- Start with general questions, such as "How may we help you today?" and work toward more probing questions. Working from simple to complex gives you time to establish rapport and builds the information background.
- Phrase your questions to require an extended response in the patient's own words, unless you need specific information. This is called *open-ended questioning* and requires that patients form answers in their own words. Closed-ended questions require brief, specific answers. (See "Getting to the Point," later in this chapter, for further discussion of these concepts.)
- Remember incongruence? Look for cues that conflict with the patient's statements of concern. What is actually bothering this patient? There may be much more to discover than the initial or presenting complaint.
- Remember that many responses are **subjective**, or obvious only to the patient; for example, pain to one patient may be discomfort to another. A small amount of blood to one patient may be hemorrhage to another. Closed-ended questions help **clarify** responses, such as exactly how much blood, or registering pain on a scale of 1 to 10 (Fig. 3-2).
- Ask one concept per question. "Do you have nausea, vomiting, and diarrhea?" may result in a positive answer when the patient has only nausea and vomiting. Patients may be too sick to separate the issues for you and will agree to whatever you say.

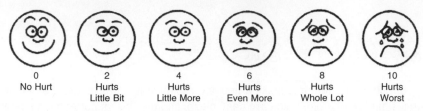

Copyright © Mosby, 2003

Figure 3-2
Example of a pain evaluation scale.
Because pain perception is subjective and varies significantly from one patient to another, pain assessment tools help make documentation reasonably simple. Although there are patients who tolerate high levels of pain with few complaints, and highly reactive patients who confuse discomfort with pain, scales such as this one help maintain a level of consistency and conformity in recording reports of pain. (Wong-Baker FACES Pain Rating Scale. In Wong DL, Hockenberry-Eaton M, Wilson D, Winkelstein ML, Schwartz P. *Wong's Essentials of Pediatric Nursing*, 6th ed. St. Louis, Mo, Mosby, 2001, p. 691.)

- Avoid "cuing" the patient's answers by your positive or negative feedback. For example, if you ask "Do you think the treatment is working?," and he answers, "No, I'm not any better," if you question again, "Are you sure?," he will presume his first response is not what you want to hear. He may change his answer to whatever he thinks you want. This is not effective, therapeutic communication and may lead to improper treatment.
- Although you must lead the line of questioning to determine the reason for the interaction, never lead the answers. For instance, "You are taking your medicine, aren't you?," probably will lead to a positive answer even if the patient stopped some time ago. A more productive **sequence** might include, "What medicines are you taking now?," followed by "How are you taking these medicines?" This type of questioning may also uncover misunderstandings as patients explain their health care routine to you. If you assume that patients are following their treatment plans correctly and simply ask for assurance that they understand what is expected, you may not discover that they do not understand important points about self-care.
- Avoid biased questions. For example, avoid a question such as, "You have never had unprotected sex, have you?" or "You have never used IV drugs, have you?" You might ask instead, "Have you ever had unprotected sex?" or "Have you ever used IV drugs?" If the answer is an emphatic "Never," the answer is more likely truthful. You have established a non-threatening, accepting attitude that lets patients know that you will not judge them for their answers (see Legal Eagle box).
- Many patients are very suggestible; if you must prompt the patient by offering leads, give him a wide range of choices. For instance, you might ask, "Mr. Martin, how long have you felt this pain?" If he answers vaguely, "I don't remember." Offer suggestions such as, "Would you say several days, two weeks, a month, or longer?" Or you may ask, "Mrs. Jones, how much blood do you think you saw: a cup, a half-cup, a tablespoon, or a teaspoon, more or less?" If your choice range is too small, patients may believe there are no other options.
- Reward patients for a productive exchange. For instance, "This is very good information. The doctor will need to know this." Patients feel they have contributed to resolving the problem.

LEGAL EAGLE

Many highly sensitive conversations regarding patients occur throughout the day in any medical setting. Remember that patient communication, treatments, diagnoses, prognoses, and other communications must never be discussed outside of the medical facility or with anyone in the facility not involved in an individual patient's care. Information may be shared only with the patient's consent and on a "need-to-know" basis. Patient information can be shared only with health care professionals directly involved in the care of the patient. Written consent is required before any information is released to anyone other than those directly involved in the patient's immediate care. Sharing information without the patient's expressed consent is illegal and may result in legal action against you.

- Indicate when the exchange is over by stressing points that need clarification and by summarizing your impressions. Ask if the patient has additional questions before moving to the next step.

Perceptive professionals can learn a lot by how patients relay information. Careful observation should help you determine what it is about the problem that is most important or causes the greatest concern. Find out what changed in the health status to cause the patient to ask for help. And, by observing cues, you may discover there is more the patient needs to tell you, but she may not know how. Remember that the **chief complaint** is only one part of the patient's problems and may not even be the main reason for asking for help. An in-depth, effective exchange brings to light all of the patient's concerns.

After building the framework for an information exchange by establishing a respectful rapport and setting a welcoming environment, asking the right questions helps gather the information needed for diagnosis and treatment with the most efficient use of time. The question styles listed below help patients organize their thoughts and relay them efficiently and effectively.

Getting to the Point

The most direct way to gather specific information is to ask questions that require patients to structure their answers. These are called open-ended questions. Encourage patients to give you answers in their own words by asking questions that include "what," "when," "where," or "how." Examples may include the following:
- "Describe <u>what</u> happened next."
- "Do you remember <u>when</u> you first felt this?"
- "Can you point to <u>where</u> it hurts?"
- "<u>How</u> did you feel when it happened?"

If possible, avoid questions asking "why?" For example, do not ask, "<u>Why</u> didn't you take your medicine?" "Why" questions seem to imply that the patient did something wrong and he may become defensive and stop trying to communicate. If you must ask "why" questions, phrase them so they do not sound like accusations.

Closed questions, or closed-ended questions, require short, direct answers for specific bits of information, such as "How many pills did you take?" or "What was the date of your last menstrual period?" This may be the information you need after a series of open-ended questions.

A combination of these types of questions usually gathers significant amounts of information.

Reflecting or Paraphrasing Responses

Open-ended statements (not questions) that repeat most of what the patient said are called **reflecting** or reflected responses. Reflected responses confirm that you received the message but leave room for more information and leave it to the patient to complete the thought or sentence. For example, you might say, "Mr. Smith, you were saying that you began to have this problem when you ....", the patient may then supply the missing information. This method encourages further comments and helps bring the patient to the point if the conversation begins to drift.

Paraphrasing repeats what the patient said using your words or phrases. This helps verify that you understood what was said. It also allows patients to clarify thoughts or statements. A paraphrased statement or question may begin, "Did I understand you to say that ...," followed by your impression of what you heard. For instance, the patient may say, "Nothing has any taste." Your response may be, "You are saying that your food does not taste as you feel it should?"

Reflecting and paraphrasing work well to gather information, but be careful not to overuse either, or some patients will wonder if you are listening.

Clarifying with Examples

Patients have as much trouble as we do making themselves understood. If you are uncertain what he is trying to tell you, ask for examples. This also may help you understand what the patient feels is the current problem and how he feels about it. For example, the patient may state, "I have felt this way for so long." You may respond, "Can you tell me about what happened and when you first noticed this feeling?"

Clarifying works both ways. We need to clarify what patients say to us and what we say to them. For example, you may need to clarify confusing statements for the patient

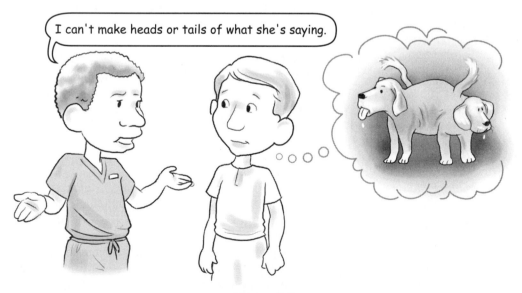

Figure 3-3

regarding medical procedures or medical terminology, not just to clear up your own confusion about what the patient said to you. Do not presume that all patients understand common medical terms or procedures. Clarifying patient instructions such as, "You are scheduled for fasting blood work today. When did you last eat or drink?" may uncover a misunderstanding about a term as common to us as fasting that could lead to serious consequences. Patients frequently misunderstand and misinterpret medical terms. Abbreviations, for example, can be very confusing. For instance, "Mr. Smith in Room 3 has SOB." We know that SOB is a common abbreviation for shortness of breath, but other patients and family members may misinterpret it as a slang phrase. Clarifying is essential for open and effective communication (Fig. 3-3).

Leading the Way

If the conversation lags, or if the patient seems to drift from the line you need to pursue, you may bring the focus back by using leads such as, "You were saying ....", or "And then what happened?" Be careful about diverting the patient from a direction he feels he needs to follow; allowing the patient to lead, within reason, may bring out information you may not have gathered in tightly focused questioning. Remember, leading the line of questions to gather specific information is not the same as asking leading questions.

Productive Silences

Silences occur in most conversations and can be a productive part of the process. However, some people are not comfortable during silences and try to fill the quiet places with words. We should use silences to form new thoughts and organize ideas, to remember events, to decide how we feel about the topic, and to summarize in our minds where we are in the conversation. Periods of silence also allow you to observe the patient quietly without dividing your attention while decoding spoken messages. Encourage silence if the patient seems particularly scattered and confused; it may be the break she needs to gather her thoughts.

Summarizing the Information

Restating and **summarizing** highlights of the information gives the patient a chance to correct himself or you, and to clarify central concerns. Use this summary to organize information into **sequential** events and to determine before you move on that you and the patient have covered every issue of concern at this time. For example, you may summarize this way, "You feel you don't have the energy recently that you usually have and that your appetite has not been good for about a month. Do I have this right?"

After establishing a proper rapport, these techniques, used appropriately, should help gather the information you need to assist the patient and the doctor toward resolving the patient's problem.

LISTENING TO WHAT YOU HEAR: IT ISN'T AS EASY AS IT SOUNDS

Listening is equally important as speaking in the transfer of information. Hearing and listening are very different concepts. *Hearing* is simply the sensory perception of sound and is usually passive. Hearing requires almost no focused involvement. *Listening*, however, means paying close attention to what we hear (Box 3-2). Active listening requires recognizing the

Box **3-2**   **How We Listen**

> Why and how do we listen? There are different forms of listening for different situations:
> - Directed—a specific transfer of information; may not require evaluation of cues
> - Attentive—gathering information for careful consideration, as in taking a medical history
> - Pleasurable—for no purpose except enjoyment; includes music and story-telling
> - Courteous—because it is the right thing to do; may not be very attentive
> - Passive—(simply hearing) sounds heard in passing and easily ignored
>
>   A patient who tries to communicate with you when you are not listening will soon give up the effort and with good reason will presume that you are not interested in his health care concerns.

significance of both verbal and nonverbal communication and involves focused perception and attentive body language on the part of the listener. Although much of what we hear does not require that we listen actively, all that we hear during patient interaction requires that we listen with close attention. As health care professionals, we must practice listening without an all-too-human tendency to filter what we hear through our preconceptions, prejudices, past experiences, and prior knowledge of the situation. An open mind and suspension of personal prejudices is vital to open communication. This issue was covered in Chapter 2, "Challenges to Communication."

In a quiet, private area, give the patient your full attention and keep interruptions and distractions to a minimum. Focus on what is being said and on what is transmitted through paralanguage, body language, and other cues. If verbal messages are incongruent with nonverbal messages, search for the reason. For example, is the patient saying she is fine, while everything you observe tells you she is not fine? If her signals are conflicting, and you cannot determine the cause, talk with the physician about your concern. You may have lost rapport with this patient if she will not open up to you and you are not able to overcome the barriers. You may have to turn her care over to another worker and review your interaction to determine why the patient is reluctant to talk to you.

We all have trouble listening at times, such as when we are far too busy and are falling behind, just at the time this patient wants and needs to ramble through his troubles. Rushed, hurried, unproductive situations are inevitable; however, active listening as a skill develops over time. These suggestions and practice will improve your listening skills, even during these difficult situations:

- Do not interpret before the patient has finished speaking. Without the full message, your interpretation may not be right and the patient may not complete the thought.
- Never complete the statement for the patient. Your conclusion may not be what he intended to say and many patients will not correct you.
- Do not spend the time the patient is speaking forming your response or your next question. You may miss valuable nonverbal cues and the patient certainly will know that you are not listening (Fig. 3-4).
- Let the patient set the speed and tone of the conversation but do gently nudge the topic toward the necessary information. Review "Leading the Way," previously in this chapter, for examples.

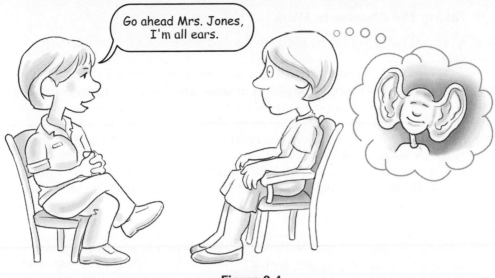

Figure 3-4

- Sit with an open posture, face-to-face and eye-to-eye. If the patient is uncomfortable with eye contact, respect his cultural needs.
- Be aware of attentive body cues, such as inclining toward the patient and using appropriate facial expressions. These cues encourage the patient to respond to you.
- Consider your responses before proceeding with questions. Decide the best way to approach this patient to gather the most complete information.
- Learn to **gate**, or exclude, sounds not involved in the exchange. Other sounds in the hallway, other voices, phones, and so on, are not your concern at this time. Tune them out and concentrate entirely on the patient (Box 3-3).

As you assist the patient to the next step of care, review your documentation. Remember that the patient's file is a legal document and your record of the interaction may be called into question. Even more important than legal protection, your part in recording information helps direct the examination or treatment, establishes a foundation of rapport, and helps put your patient at ease.

Box **3-3**   **Creating a Sound Barrier**

As you sit in your classroom, you are surrounded by sound, even during the enforced quiet of an examination . . . papers rattle, pens scratch, feet shuffle under desks, sounds continue in the hallway. If you concentrate on what you are doing, you can gate these sounds and choose not to hear them. You may not be aware of this skill, but you use it any time you exclude or diminish all the sounds around you except the one most important to you. Develop this skill; learn to ignore every sound in the health care setting not directly related to this patient's immediate care. This skill is the foundation of focused interaction.

Taking the Chapter to Work

Now, let's meet Patsy and see how she has applied this chapter information in the workplace.

Patsy is working in an orthopedic clinic. She has begun to interview a patient who is 84 years old and has multiple complaints of aches and pains. The patient has been seen in the clinic on multiple occasions for arthritis. Patsy starts by asking the patient open-ended questions using the words "what," "where," "when," and "how." The patient states that she has had aches and pains for years. Patsy then clarifies this information by asking "The aches and pains in your knees started at the same time as the aches in your back. Is that correct?" The patient states that the knee pains have been present for years, but the back pain started two days ago and that is why she made today's appointment. Patsy then directs her questioning about the back pain and finds out that the patient also has had trouble urinating and is experiencing burning and itching sensations after voiding. Patsy identifies these signs as a possible urinary tract infection and communicates this to the physician. A urinary specimen is obtained, and it shows signs of an infection.

Because Patsy took the time to clarify and reflect on the patient's answers, she was able to identify the root of today's problem. It is important to explore all patient complaints and search for possible problems and not allow yourself to become complacent.

Beyond the Classroom Exercises

Your Assignment Board

The following exercises will help you apply what you learned in the chapter. Place a check beside the assignments your instructor has given you. When you have completed the assignment, place a check in the completed column.

		Assigned	*Completed*
Checking Your Comprehension	(Textbook)	☐	☐
Expanded Critical Thinking	(Textbook)	☐	☐
Communication Surfer Exercises	(Textbook and Internet)	☐	☐
Communication Tree Branch #3	(CD-ROM)	☐	☐
Communication Tree Branch #4	(CD-ROM)	☐	☐
Voice Mail Message #3	(CD-ROM)	☐	☐
Health History Chart	(CD-ROM)	☐	☐
Patient/Caregiver Interview #1	(CD-ROM)	☐	☐
Patient/Caregiver Interview #2	(CD-ROM)	☐	☐

 ### Checking Your Comprehension

Write a brief answer for each of the following assignments.
1. Define an algorithm and explain its purpose.
2. Explain the difference between an open-ended and a closed-ended question and give two examples of each type.
3. Define *acronym* and give two examples.
4. Explain the difference between the terms *paraphrasing* and *reflecting*. Tell why each is important. Give an example of each.
5. Explain the benefit of allowing silences during a patient interview.
6. Explain the difference between *hearing* and *listening*. Discuss why listening is so important.

Expanding Critical Thinking

1. The following patients all have symptoms of nausea and vomiting. List five questions you would ask each of these patients or family members. How are your questions different in each situation? Which questions are common to all patients?
   a. A mother reporting about her 1-week-old son, or her 3-year-old daughter, or her 9-year-old son. (Choose one or more of the children in different age groups. Compare and contrast the types of questions you should ask.)
   b. A 20-year-old woman with no other symptoms and normal vital signs.
   c. An elderly woman with sharp pains in her upper right abdomen and stable vital signs.
   d. A chronic alcoholic with obvious jaundice and stable vital signs.
   e. An otherwise-healthy 30-year-old athletic man with a temperature of 102° F.

Continued

Expanding Critical Thinking—Cont'd

2. Create an algorithm of questions for two different patient complaints of your choice.
3. Create an acronym for two different patient complaints of your choice.
4. Which of the methods in Questions 2 and 3 works best for you in the interview process? Why?
5. Reread the Legal Eagle box. All patient conversations are confidential; however, some situations are more sensitive and personal than others. List five such topics. Are you comfortable questioning patients about these topics? If the answer is "no," which ones bother you and why? How can you overcome your reluctance to talk about these issues?
6. Silence makes some people uncomfortable. How do you feel about silence during a conversation? Experiment with a family member or fellow student. How did he or she feel? How did you feel?
7. Can you gate successfully? How can you improve your ability to eliminate distractions?
8. Determine whether stress affects your ability to gate. When you are tired and still need to study, do you find that overheard conversations and noisy distractions are harder or easier to gate? Are you more or less irritated at interruptions when you are stressed?
9. As you question Mrs. Brown about her current concern, she gives you answers that do not make sense. She lives alone and drives herself where she needs to go, but you suspect her orientation and reasoning are impaired. What should you do?

 Communication Surfer Exercises

1. Reread the Legal Eagle box. It states that "written consent" is required before information is released. Using the Internet, locate sites for the American Hospital Association (AHA) and the Joint Commission on Accreditation for Hospitals (JCAHO). Both of these organizations have recommendations for consent forms. What items should be included in a consent form?
2. Before you can communicate effectively with a patient, the patient's pain must be managed. Using the Internet for research, create a list of 10 ways that you could help a patient control pain without the use of medications. Then search the Internet for types of pain medications. Make a list of 10 prescription pain medications. By using the Internet, learn the common side effects generally associated with pain medications. How could these side effects affect your ability to communicate with a patient?

4

EDUCATING PATIENTS: TEACHING PATIENTS TO HELP THEMSELVES

LEARNING OBJECTIVES

Upon successfully completing this chapter, you will be able to:

- Explain your role in patient education.
- Outline the information you need before you begin to teach.
- List and describe factors that make teaching and learning more difficult.
- List and describe factors that make teaching and learning easier.
- Research appropriate teaching plan resources for a variety of situations.
- Prepare an effective teaching and evaluation plan for specific situations.

KEY TERMS

Adherence
Affective
Assess, assessment
Cognitive
Document, documenting, documentation

Evaluate, evaluation
Estranged
Holistic
Implement, implementation
Learning goal
Learning objectives

Noncompliance
Patient education
Planning
Psychomotor

Test Your Communication IQ

Before reading this chapter, complete this short self-assessment test. Decide which statements are true and which are false.

1. If a patient asks you a question that you cannot answer, it is best to guess at an answer so you communicate to the patient that you are a knowledgeable, experienced, and qualified professional.
2. Too much information at once is confusing; smaller, more manageable sessions are easier to understand and retain.
3. Imagined pain or the perception of pain can hurt as much as pain with a physical origin.
4. Support group facilitators must help motivate the group, coordinate, and schedule the meetings, and should encourage a broad range of discussion from all group members.
5. Patients should be discouraged from using the Internet for patient education.
6. Italic lettering is recommended when creating patient education booklets to present a pleasing format.

Results

Statements two and three are true; all others statements are false. How did you do? Read the chapter to learn more about the topics.

M ost **patient education** involves helping patients return to the best possible state of health after an acute illness. If a full return to wellness is not possible, patients may need help learning to live with chronic conditions. However, much of our effort in health care should be directed at keeping patients well before illnesses have a chance to develop. In Chapter 5, "Communicating Wellness," we will learn health care factors our patients need to know to restore or maintain health. Your clinical manuals cover information regarding performance skills that you and your patient need to correct or manage the outcome of many illnesses and will be the basis of much of your teaching. You will find, though, that all of this information and all of your skills combined will not benefit the patient once he is home and no longer under your care if he does not understand his part in correcting or maintaining health. One of our major health care duties is to educate patients and caregivers in the proper means of retaining or restoring health. To that purpose, this chapter covers how to transmit information to a variety of patients in a manner best suited to their individual needs.

To help control the increasing cost of health care, hospitals discharge patients earlier and with greater medical needs now than in years past. As much as 90% of post-hospital care will be self-care or home care, involving ongoing treatments, medications, and lifestyle changes monitored by the patient or his caregivers, frequently with only occasional oversight by medical professionals. These sick patients and their caregivers need more help from health educators and more direction from their health care providers to ensure that health maintenance plans are understood and followed. This requires that the patient and caregivers understand as fully as possible what must be done to achieve health care goals.

The purposes of educating the patient in self-care are as follows:

- To promote, maintain, and restore health.
- To raise the standard of health.
- To help the patient cope with the lasting effects of illness.

LEGAL EAGLE

It is very important to work within your scope of practice guidelines. Exceeding your scope of practice or level of responsibility can put your career in jeopardy and can endanger your patients. In certain cases, you may lose your license or certificate, be fined, or even terminated from your position. If you are unsure of your scope of practice and responsibility in patient education or other tasks, communicate your concerns to your supervisor for clarification.

Many agencies employ health educators to oversee and coordinate patient teaching, but every member of the team is responsible for reinforcing the patient's understanding of how to maintain or regain a reasonable level of health. Changing a dressing, assisting with procedures, and administering medications have a more visible effect, and may be more immediately rewarding to you and the patient, but patient education has a longer lasting effect on overall health. Patient education is as important as any clinical responsibility that you perform. Each member of the team is expected to treat patient teaching as seriously as any other clinical duty and must never miss an opportunity to reinforce good health habits (see the Legal Eagle box).

MAKING SURE YOUR PATIENT LEARNS

Education and compliance work best if the approach centers on the patient's **holistic** needs. These include spiritual, physical, emotional, social, and economic needs, not just medical needs. For example, consider how disruptive an illness and its treatments will be to all areas of the patient's life. How expensive is the treatment, and at what sacrifice? Will he be able to work at his chosen career? Can she continue to care for her family? Will the illness become debilitating, or is it manageable with lifestyle changes? What is this patient's cultural concepts of the illness, its cause, and traditional medicine's cures? Patients must trust health care providers to know these things, to have their best interests at heart, and to involve them in decisions about the direction of care that may profoundly affect the rest of their lives.

We will find as we work toward educating patients that we value the "good" patient, one who complies with all we suggest, who does not question, who does not complain, and who passively follows any health care plan set for him, either for correction or prevention. Unfortunately, we frequently resent the "difficult" patient who makes independent health care choices. This does not include patients who will not follow health care plans and then wonder why their health does not improve. These "difficult" patients ask questions regarding their care, make suggestions that differ from ours, and make logical and healthful changes that work better for them than those we suggest. Although this may annoy those of us who presume we know best, this is actually the goal of health care and more likely leads to a healthy lifestyle than the behavior of a patient who blindly follows directions without questions or understanding. The "difficult" patient may be the most compliant, because he feels he has an active part in his care. He understands and agrees to the needed treatment, asks questions, and monitors his treatment to be sure it has the expected results. He knows that most of his wellness is under his control.

As you work toward determining your patient's health education needs, also consider your feelings about the patient and the illness. If you are uncomfortable talking with the patient about some factor in health care prevention or treatment, discuss this with the physician. You may need someone to take your place on the health care team. It is unrealistic to presume that you will never come across situations that make you uncomfortable or that are offensive to you. If this happens, and you cannot set aside or overcome your discomfort, you owe it to your patients to turn over their care to someone else. If you are prejudiced against the patient or the illness, or simply uncomfortable in the situation, you may find it difficult to keep the patient's best interest foremost in the interaction. If your patient senses your discomfort, effective communication may not be possible.

In addition, determine how well you know the information or how skilled you are at performing a required procedure. If you are unsure of anything you are responsible for teaching, ask someone to walk you through the steps or read all available information before you begin. Patients count on you to know as much as you can about factors affecting their health, and you owe it to yourself and your professionalism to present a credible presence to your patients. If your patient asks you a question that you cannot answer, be honest and explain, "I don't know the answer, but I will find out and will let you know." If you create an answer that is wrong, not only will you lose your professional credibility, the misinformation may actually harm the patient.

When you have your information in place, begin the education process. Patient education involves these five steps:

- Assessment
- Planning
- Implementation
- Evaluation
- Documentation

Each of these steps is equally important in effective patient teaching.

Determining Your Patient's Learning Style

Looking at all factors in any situation is called **assessment** and is the first step in most health care interaction. Consider points such as these when determining, or assessing, the patient's current educational needs: Is she emotionally and physically able to absorb possibly complex concepts? Is she too nauseated or sedated to listen and learn? How acute are his senses? Can he see you? Can he hear you? If English is his second language, can he understand you? Are you speaking beyond her level of education? Is he motivated to learn? Is she emotionally ready to learn, or is she still in denial? Has he accepted his illness and the consequences? Is she ready to assume responsibility for her own care and return to health? How much does he understand about his health care issues? How does she feel about the effects of this illness on her future? How much experience has he had with the health care system to this point? What is her medical and surgical history? Is it extensive, implying long-term involvement in health care, or is it brief, alerting you that she may not understand how to work through the medical system? The process is easier and more productive if you understand the patient's physical and emotional needs before deciding how to approach health care education.

Determining how much the patient already knows and understands about the illness can direct how much and what type of information is needed in each situation. For example, diabetics who do not understand the fundamentals of nutrition will not understand or retain information as well as those already actively involved in good dietary habits. Patients with a poor nutritional background may require a referral to a nutritionist or dietitian to help establish a working foundation. Likewise, a patient who understands exercise physiology will more likely continue a physical therapy routine than one who is set in an inactive lifestyle. Learning is easier when we already have an established knowledge base for adding new information.

You may know most of the patient's background information, such as sensory barriers, education and comprehension levels, and so forth, from previous interaction with the patient or from the record. Consult other staff members and the patient's caregivers for additional information that will make education easier.

Next, determine the patient's best style of learning. These include the following:

- **Cognitive**—processing facts, forming conclusions, and making decisions by listening to or reading instructions or information. Most literate adults do well with self-directed, independent learning when they understand how important it is, especially if they feel that the learning experience is under their control. Most patients quickly and easily understand that learning how to handle an illness will help improve their health or, at the very least, help them cope with the changes they are experiencing. For example, many well-educated, assertive patients research their illnesses and will approach you with stacks of information from many sources, some more reliable than others. They may even challenge you with information they find that contradicts what you are trying to teach. If the information gathered by patients disagrees with agency policy, let the physician know so that more time can be set aside to explain the purpose of the individual treatment plan.

- **Affective**—appealing to emotions or feelings to change someone's beliefs or attitude and reinforce the importance of the change in concepts. It is more difficult to learn new information if it goes against firmly held beliefs. However, once adults are convinced it is important to their health, most will adapt to new concepts. The new way of thinking and believing may need to be explained or approached from different viewpoints and by various means until the patient accepts the information. This may include recruiting family members to help convince the patient of its importance, or introducing patients to support groups of those who have experienced the same type of health problem with a positive outcome. For example, a woman who believes that she will no longer be a desirable mate if she has a hysterectomy or mastectomy may need to speak with someone from a support group who has experienced her same doubts and fears. If she can believe that she will still be desirable, she will more likely change her mind and her beliefs. She may not agree to the surgery until she can accept that the changes in her body image will not interfere with forming and maintaining relationships.

- **Psychomotor**—learning by doing, as in demonstration of a skill. If the new knowledge can be taught by active participation in a skill, understanding is more likely for those who learn best by doing. For example, your patient may accept the need to learn how to self-inject his insulin and may have read what he needs to know, but until he has practiced the steps with you, you cannot be sure that he understands not only how to do it right, but what may happen if he does it wrong.

Most people have one learning method they prefer, but we all learn best by combining all three methods. This helps store information in more areas of our brain for better recall. The more places we store information (seeing, hearing, reading, reasoning, doing), the better we remember. To retain information, we must receive data, compare it to what we already know, store it in accessible memory banks, and value the information enough to keep it for future reference, much as a computer does for future use. We remember best those things we know are important. And we remember most easily those things that relate to something we already know and can add to our knowledge base.

When you have gathered all you need to know and to relay to the patient, start the next step of the education process.

Planning for Learning

Proper and effective **planning** for education includes all information gathered during the interview and assessment process and ideally involves the whole health care team. For example, an education plan for a newly diagnosed patient with diabetes may require input from an endocrinologist, a dietitian, a home health service representative, and the coordinating physician. After a stroke, a patient may need assistance from the primary care physician, a neurologist, a physical therapist, and a speech therapist. All of this coordination of services must consider what patients need to know and do, but planning for care should also involve patients in the necessary decisions. We are all more likely to comply with suggestions and directions if we feel involved in making decisions that affect us. Patients have a feeling of control if they are allowed to create schedules, learn new performance skills, or adopt lifestyle changes that consider their likes and dislikes and their preferences and limitations, while still following medical protocol. This makes them participants in the return to health. No one appreciates being told what to do with no input or consideration for personal needs.

Planning should include a definable goal. Learning goals and objectives must be defined with expected short-term and long-term results. **Learning goals** outline the desired results of the educational program. **Learning objectives** include procedures or tasks to be discussed or performed at various points in the program. Objectives and goals should be created specifically for each patient and each situation and must include a standard by which learning and achievement can be measured (Teaching Plan box).

For example, consider the patient who must learn to distinguish between angina pectoris and a myocardial infarction. Which of these objectives is more specific and allows a measurement of progress?

• Patient and caregiver will understand how to manage acute angina pectoris.
• Patient and caregiver will demonstrate sufficient knowledge of cardiovascular function and dysfunction to recognize signs of impending myocardial infarction and to identify proper preventive and corrective measures.

The second plan outlines the patient's and caregiver's responsibility and, if psychomotor skills are required, ideally should include step-by-step procedures such as those you use in clinical proficiencies. A checklist works well if the patient forgets a step, or wonders what comes next. Just as your proficiency checklist keeps your performance in line, this sort of self-care aid also works for patients.

Patients who receive instructions for physician-approved treatment plans and patient education material (PEM) must sign that they received it and understand it. Copies with the patient's signature should be kept in the patient's record. The original is given to the patient. Documenting the education process and the patient's understanding is covered in the Teaching Plan box.

TEACHING PLAN

FOR A PATIENT WITH ONSET OF ACUTE ANGINA PECTORIS

Learning Objectives: Patient and caregiver will demonstrate sufficient knowledge of cardiovascular function and dysfunction to practice appropriate preventive measures and to recognize signs of impending myocardial infarction and initiate corrective measures.

Learning Goal: Patient and caregiver will understand and practice prudent lifestyle changes for an improvement in cardiovascular functioning and decrease in high-risk cardiovascular factors.

Teaching Plan	Criteria for Evaluation
Evaluate patient and caregiver readiness and motivation to learn	Patient and caregiver will prepare a list of questions regarding cardiovascular functions and dysfunction and the need for prudent living for review with staff
Assess patient and caregiver knowledge base and deficits	Patient and caregiver will discuss their concept of cardiovascular disease, its prevention, and treatment with staff
Determine the preferred learning style and literacy level of patient and caregiver	Health care worker will consult with physician regarding best method for patient education
Provide specific PEM at the appropriate literacy level outlining warning signs of angina pectoris versus myocardial infarction and what to do for both	Patient and caregiver will compile a list of checkpoints for comparison and an algorithm for 911 contact
Review medication regimen and supply written explanations and directions for each	Patient and caregiver will explain benefits and adverse reactions for each medication and list the dosage schedule
Determine understanding of medication regimen by having patient and caregiver restate in own words or demonstrate proficiency	Health care worker will rate understanding of patient and caregiver explanation and demonstration of medication regimen proficiency
Determine that caregiver has completed CPR course	"Friends and Family CPR" course completion card
Review patient and caregiver emergency plan if angina pectoris is not resolved and myocardial infarction is suspected	Review written plan or algorithm for emergency care

This information was explained to me to my understanding.

_____   _____
　　　　　(patient)   (caregiver)

Comments: _____

_____

Implementing the Process

Implementation puts the process in motion and can be carried out in several ways to suit the patient's needs. You may instruct patients through one-on-one or group discussion, or by teaching aids such as videos and audiocassettes, or take-home references such as booklets, pamphlets, or brochures. Call on other members of the health care team or community support group members to help as needed during this process.

After determining how your patient prefers to learn, you can choose any of the following proven implementation methods.

Lecture and demonstration present the basic information but do not require participation to reinforce or retain the information. In this format, information is relayed and procedures are performed without the patient's participation. This may be enough for highly motivated patients who you know are generally compliant, but it does not work well for patients who need to participate in learning by psychomotor, or hands-on, reinforcement. Written information should be available for reference if questions come up later, and patients should know they can call to clear up misunderstandings when they have had time to think back over all they have learned.

Role-playing and demonstration require that you perform a medical procedure as the patient watches, then the patient performs it so that you can **evaluate** his or her understanding. Patients who actively participate in the process of learning are more likely to retain the information.

When you demonstrate procedures for patients to perform at home, make examples as realistic as possible so that patients can anticipate how to perform them correctly during in-home care. Patients generally do not have homes in any way like the medical setting and have to work through bathrooms, kitchens, or other places not at all like the setting in which they were instructed. Those who do not understand important points, or who cannot translate what they learned into their home environment, may delay recovery or may make the situation worse rather than better.

Psychomotor skills are easier to learn if you demonstrate the skill first, explaining each step as you perform it for the patient, then have the patient perform each step with your support or assistance. Finally, have the patient work through the process without your help until you feel the level of skill is appropriate for self-care. Even with the best of demonstrations, written instructions should be available for reference as needed. Skills checklists work well at this point for reinforcement.

Discussion is a back-and-forth exchange of information and concepts and works best for education regarding lifestyle changes but does not work well for medical procedures. In this format, you present information and patients relay back to you what they understand and how this affects them. This reinforces affective or emotional retention of information.

Discussion can be one-on-one, or may be conducted as a group. A combination of both works best. Patients who are confident and assertive do well in either format but may dominate the discussion and exclude those less able to express themselves; quiet patients may be lost in a group environment. Be alert for cues from any group situation if you suspect that less assertive members are being overlooked and their concerns neglected as the group concentrates on patients who are more vocal. This requires tact and diplomacy on your part to avoid offending any member of the group.

Group dynamics and working with support groups are covered later in this chapter in "The Importance of Support Groups."

Audio-visual material works well for those who are not motivated to read, but you must have a method for determining how well the patient understands the information contained in the material. Go over the information with the patient and ask appropriate questions to check for understanding. Having patients explain to you in their own terms what they understood is more likely to bring out misunderstandings than simply asking if he or she understands the information. Patients may take the material home to review as needed. Videos to use at home reinforce skills and concepts taught in the medical setting and are reassuring to patients who may have trouble remembering all of the steps in an involved procedure, even with a checklist.

An interesting and very personal aid involves a video of yourself and the patient as you work through the steps of a procedure. If this is possible in your facility, patients find videos of themselves far more interesting than those of anonymous actors performing the same tasks; therefore, they are more likely to review the tape frequently.

Printed material and programmed instructions can be covered with patients to discuss and clarify points and to bring out questions they may have before presuming they understand the information. These materials are available from many sources and are covered in "Choosing and Adapting Teaching Materials" later in this chapter. Physicians must review all material and teaching methods to ensure the information is appropriate for each patient's needs and that it follows the practices and philosophies of the facility.

Previous chapters alerted you to cues that a patient may have trouble understanding complex concepts. Many evaluation tools are available to determine literacy levels and are covered later in this chapter; however, if you suspect that your patient cannot read well, try using visual and verbal education methods, repeat the instructions as often as needed, use different levels of language skills, and watch for cues indicating the patient understands. Have the patient repeat the instructions back to you. Diagrams and pictures help for nonreading patients. If medical concepts are beyond the patient's comprehension, ask the patient's caregiver to work with you. If you suspect that neither the patient nor the caregiver understands what you are trying to teach, alert the physician; a home health agency may need to be involved until everyone feels comfortable with the situation.

After deciding which combination of the formats listed above works best in each situation, use all of the appropriate communication skills you have learned to transmit the information. These suggestions will help reinforce the learning experience:

- Keep up with current medical advances and make sure the information available in your agency is up-to-date. Many of our patients are well informed and appreciate receiving appropriate information from their health care professionals. Patients less involved in their own care and who are unlikely to look for information, such as in journals and on Internet sites, need you to provide and interpret emerging medical technology for them.
- With the physician's permission, help patients and caregivers contact appropriate support groups. Most support groups provide books, brochures, and videos, and compile lists of local resources for assistance in dealing with Alzheimer's patients, colostomy care, postmastectomy recovery, and so on.
- Help patients find community resources to continue complicated at-home care; these include home health agencies, medical supply companies, and so forth. Many pharmaceutical and medical supply companies have well-written information regarding how to use their products and are eager to share this information for patient education.
- Build on the patient's knowledge base—what does she already know about what you need to teach?—and add new information in a simple-to-complex sequence.

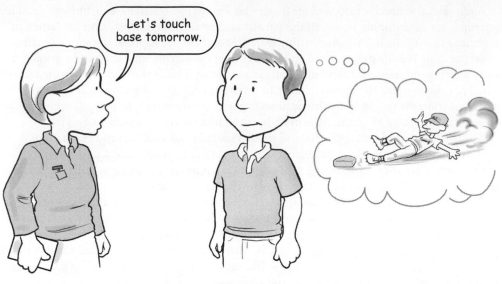

Figure 4-1

- Allow time for questions and clarification. Patients who feel rushed may not have time to absorb the information and may be too confused and overwhelmed to think of appropriate questions.
- When checking for comprehension, rather than asking, "Did you understand what we just covered?", ask specific points such as, "Can you tell me when you should use Standard Precautions?" and "How will you dispose of your soiled dressings?" Answers to these open-ended questions are more revealing, since they require more of the patient than "yes" or "no."
- Offer to call patients in the next day or so to check for additional questions or concerns (Fig. 4-1). Patients who are hesitant and unsure of themselves may be reluctant to call you with what may seem at first a small problem, which then can become a much larger health issue if not corrected in a timely manner.
- Be available for questions and concerns; this helps to reevaluate goals and objectives that are not working.
- Arrange for visits as needed to the health care facility for evaluation and additional education as needed. Home health agencies are available to reinforce at-home care if the patient does not need to return to your agency or if transportation is a problem.

With proper teaching methods in place, the patient and his caregivers should be ready now to perform health care away from medical supervision.

Evaluating the Goals

Determining the patient's progress and continued understanding of medical care plans is part of the education process. Evaluations of understanding and progress are made frequently in the hospital setting with constant contact. However, when the patient is responsible for self-care and contact is limited, the patient or caregiver must evaluate progress and report to someone responsible for coordinating care. Working with the physician and patient, you can help plan a convenient and appropriate schedule for progress reports. If the patient does not contact you or the agency by a predetermined schedule, it is your responsibility to check to determine how well the patient is progressing. If you find that he or she did not understand the care plan, or is not complying, the health care team needs to determine why. Did she understand how compliance affects her health? Is he committed to whatever it takes to get well? The team may need to schedule more in-depth education and evaluation if the patient is not following the care plan. If the care plan is too complicated or difficult, a home health agency should be contacted to help with home care. Making it easier to comply with treatment plans increases the chances of finding good results during evaluation.

If the treatment plan involves a procedure, observe the patient performing the steps at different times during her care. If she is doing it correctly, praise her and encourage her efforts. If the patient is not performing the procedure correctly, tactfully, without making her feel inferior, guide her in the correct performance. A performance checklist helps prevent missed steps. Many patients gradually become less compliant as time goes by; therefore, frequent evaluations may be needed to make sure the patient continues to follow the plan and to evaluate the need for changes in procedures as the patient improves or the illness progresses.

If specific information needs to be documented, such as amount and type of wound drainage or blood glucose levels, be sure the patient understands what to report and how to describe it. Be specific regarding what you mean by large amounts, small amounts, sizes, relative values, and so on, all of which are confusing to patients who wonder, "Should I report this or not?" Urge patients to call with any concerns; be receptive and understand that what looks like a small amount of anything to us may be quite a large amount for patients not used to seeing blood and body fluids (particularly their own), or dealing with complicated monitoring devices that flash confusing numbers. Always praise patients for reporting anything that causes concern, otherwise they may be reluctant to report something that may become a major health care issue.

Use short-term goals with positive feedback to encourage patients to continue to progress. For example, "Mr. Jones, you have done a good job keeping your dressing clean. The wound looks good. Now it is time to begin to soak the area." Too much information at once is confusing to patients who are adjusting to too many new concepts and procedures to grasp even one more instruction. Break complicated information into smaller steps. Unless the need-to-know is pressing at this time, wait until the next contact to teach the next step.

Evaluation may be informal and casual. For example, to evaluate dietary compliance, casually ask about lunch today or dinner last evening. You may be surprised by what you learn. To determine if the patient understands the significance of glucose levels, casually remark, "Your glucose level is 164. What do you think that means?" If this is done in a non-judgmental manner, she may explain her misconceptions about how food affects her glucose level, giving you the perfect teaching moment. Document casual exchanges just as you would more formal and structured evaluations.

Learning goals and objectives need to be reevaluated and restructured as the patient progresses through treatment. Is the health care problem resolving naturally, or is the patient's health deteriorating? Are there other changes in the patient's status that require adjustment of the goals and objectives? Is there advanced technology or a new theory that applies to the patient's situation? Yesterday's plans frequently must be altered to fit today's needs. Plan from the beginning to fit flexibility into patient education as situations change, and continue throughout the process to evaluate how well the plan is working.

Do not forget to evaluate your efforts at education. How do you think you handled the situation? What went right or wrong? How can you improve next time? How the patient learns is only part of the education equation; how you teach is equally important.

Documenting the Results

Documenting health care is vitally important in maintaining continuity of care, ensuring quality of care, and providing a legal record of care. No well-trained health care professional would give an injection and then neglect to document the medication. Patient education is equally important in restoring and maintaining patients' health. In health care, it is presumed that any service that is not documented was not performed; this, of course, includes patient education. Each step of the education process must be documented and should include the following:

- The date and time of the session if separate from regular care, such as over the phone. Include education given during routine patient care under the appropriate record entry.
- The method used, such as discussion, videos, or demonstrations.
- The information covered, such as Standard Precautions during dressing changes, glucose monitoring, dietary restriction, and so forth.
- A copy of the signed educational material provided to the patient when appropriate. The patient keeps the original and signs that the information has been explained adequately.
- Your evaluation of the patient's comprehension.
- The next scheduled evaluation for education and compliance updates.

At the end of each education session, each worker involved should sign the record to document the extent of material covered and his or her qualifications as a health care professional. If interpreters for patients who speak English as a second language were included in the process, or if the education included caregivers, document this information also.

As you evaluate understanding and compliance, remember to record each contact. This includes telephone contact with either the patient or caregiver and not simply face-to-face contact. Even casual conversations with patients or caregivers that result in insight into patient care should be recorded.

IS YOUR PATIENT READY TO LEARN?

To "learn" is defined as "To gain knowledge, comprehension, or mastery through experience or study; to fix in the mind or memorize; to acquire experience, ability or skill" (*American Heritage Dictionary*). All of our patient education goals are directed toward increasing the patient's knowledge, understanding, and mastery of the information needed to return to health, to maintain health, or to cope with the effects of illness. To do this, we must make learning as easy as possible by determining how to help the patient understand and retain the necessary information.

Think about how you learn. What factors in your life affect your ability to learn, either by promoting or by hindering it? Once you identify these factors, you know how to strengthen the good ones, eliminate the bad ones, or cope with ones you cannot change. Use this same strategy when dealing with the factors that affect patient learning.

Most patient teaching is fairly informal. Patients usually are not sitting in a classroom prepared to learn with a textbook and pen and paper. Many of your opportunities to teach are on-the-spot questions from your patients that indicate a need to know and, equally important, a desire to learn. These are called "educable moments." If patients or caregivers ask a question, seize the moment and answer every question to the best of your ability, or refer them to the proper person if you do not know the answers. Other spur-of-the-moment situations involve directions from the physician to "Show Mr. Jones how to ...." or "Tell Mrs. Smith what she needs to know about ...." In all of these situations, gather the information you need in the appropriate form (booklets, brochures, videos), observe all communication cues and factors affecting comprehension, and document the exchange when you feel that you have covered the material for this session. Unless you and the patient were prepared for an education session, it may be best to cover only small amounts of need-to-know information at this time and have the patient return for follow-up evaluations and further education when you have time to prepare for a more formal and in-depth explanation of the material.

Whether your patient is ready to learn usually is decided during the determination or assessment phase outlined above. Always offer and take advantage of opportunities for patient education, but if the patient is resistant today, or simply not prepared or motivated to learn, much of the information will be forgotten or misunderstood, which can be frustrating for both of you.

Points and questions to consider in determining readiness include the following:

- What is her energy level today? Is she free from pain, sedation, nausea? It is easier to communicate and educate without interference from physical factors.
- Is he too stressed? You may need to schedule another appointment later, unless the information is immediately important. Give him the information he needs today, and when he has adjusted to his new status, have him come back and bring a list of questions for a more formal and extensive education session.
- Is she motivated and ready to learn today? Does she still see all of this information and new way of life as too depressing, expensive, intrusive, or overwhelming? Until patients are ready to learn, limit education to the most important information on a need-to-know-now basis.
- Does he realize that learning this information is important? If he doesn't value the information, he will not retain it. We remember best those things we consider important. If you explain to him the importance of this medication, but he knows that it has severe side effects and is very expensive, he may prefer not to take it. In that case, not only will he not learn what he needs to know about the medication and his condition, he probably will not comply with other care plans pertaining to this illness.
- If much of the care will fall on the patient's caregiver, is he or she with the patient today? Educating patients who will not be responsible for their own care may be frustrating for both of you, and the lessons must be repeated later for the caregiver.

What Makes Learning Difficult?

Many factors interfere with a patient's ability to learn what we need to teach. We speak a medical language foreign to most of our patients, and we use terms that are frightening because of their reflection of the patient's health. We do strange, usually painful procedures that "normal" people usually do not do. We know their most intimate secrets and may have seen them at their very worst. In most cases, patient education follows news that may have a profound and possibly long-term effect on the patient's future. This is not the best atmosphere for learning.

Read over Chapter 2, "Challenges to Communication," for suggestions to eliminate, or at least reduce, as many barriers as possible and consider the following:

- Patients who are overwhelmed by pain, sedation, or emotional shock cannot learn. Relieve as many of these factors as possible and proceed when the patient is ready.
- Patients who use sensory aids, such as hearing aids or glasses, must have them in place before they can fully understand what you are saying or demonstrating.
- Trying to educate a patient in a hospital bed or on an examining table in a paper gown puts him at a disadvantage. If possible, wait until the patient feels more in control and presentable before beginning an education session.
- If you are not prepared with proper teaching tools, or are unsure of the information, wait if possible until you have the necessary knowledge and educational material before you begin.
- If the patient does not speak English well, and you do not have an interpreter, the attempts at communication will be frustrating for both of you.

Socioeconomic and educational backgrounds are very important in learning. If the patient feels he has never had control over the major factors in his life, he may be passive now and may not ask questions. If she is well educated and has a good self-concept, she will be more comfortable asking clarifying questions, she has a better knowledge base, and is better at seeking self-help. Those who are best at seeking help for themselves have more control over their health and usually do best at self-care. Unfortunately, those who need more help are frequently the least able or likely to ask for it.

During the determination or assessment phase, consider the potential factors that promote and hinder learning before teaching even begins. However, you can use the suggestions listed above at any time you feel the patient education process is not working.

Maslow's Hierarchy of Needs

Patients have trouble complying with patient education and probably cannot learn if certain basic needs are not met. This concept was introduced in the late 1960s by an American psychiatrist named Abraham Maslow. Maslow developed the theory that we move through areas of basic human needs that are necessary for a healthy existence before we can progress to higher needs and personal accomplishment. The highest need includes a desire to learn. Maslow determined that a need is essential if,

- Without its fulfillment or presence, illness results.
- Fulfilling the need restores homeostasis or wellness.
- We feel a sense of satisfaction when the need is met.

Maslow designed a pyramid to illustrate his concept, with the most basic needs at the base and the highest attainments at the apex, or highest point. He taught that we cannot work to fill a higher need until the earlier needs or steps have been met or satisfied. Read Box 4-1 and consider how the needs apply to your patients.

The Noncompliant Patient

Why would a patient go through making an appointment or checking into a hospital, submit to humiliating personal questions in what seems to be a foreign language, be poked, probed, and inspected by virtual strangers, give up blood and body fluid, pay for all of this, and then not comply with patient education to ensure his health? It may not be that he cannot learn; it may be that he simply chooses not to learn.

Box **4-1**   **Maslow's Hierarchy**

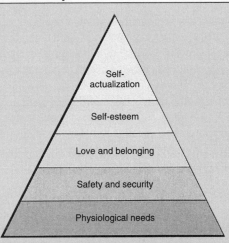

Starting at the most basic step, Maslow illustrated human needs as follows.

Physiological needs are essential for life and are the basis on which all else depends. These include oxygen, water, nourishment, proper temperature, elimination, and rest balanced with activity. Think how these most basic needs, if not met, interfere with patient education. If the patient cannot breathe, if she is thirsting, starving, too cold or overheated, in pain, or is sleep-deprived, how likely is she to listen and learn until these needs are met? Many of these needs are barriers to communication in health care.

Safety and security include shelter, adequate food, financial security, freedom from fear, and a strong support group. In America, we value our independence and form more loosely woven networks than societies that value interdependency; however, we still need to trust that we will be safe when we need protection. Consider how this need may be affected by war, famine, or natural disasters. Think of the abused wife who fears for her life but who has just discovered a lump in her breast. She may be more concerned with the probability of further abuse than the possibility of cancer. Or consider the family with small children living in a car or in the streets. They are aware that children need childhood immunizations, but health care is not their most pressing need. Until safety and security needs are met, health care, particularly preventive care, is a low priority. Children are especially susceptible to fear from loss of security and usually respond better to the medical setting if parents participate in their care to reinforce this basic need.

Love and belonging means family for most people, but also may mean a strong support group or community network. Without someone to care for us, we feel isolated and depressed and are less likely to care whether we follow prudent living standards. Since this level is closely aligned with the preceding step, filling this need may give us the safety and security we crave. This is evident in dangerous communities that foster gangs; members belong and are valued as they offer and receive protection within the group. This is seen also in countries without America's general level of safety. Cultures in these situations band together for protection from anyone outside the group, for safety and security as well as for belonging. Health care directives are less likely to be followed if they oppose cultural traditions and separate our patients from their groups, or prevent them from being full, active members. Since all formal groups have rituals and standards, health care instructions that go against the traditions of the group push the patient back to a lower level of needs fulfillment.

Continued

Box **4-1**   **Maslow's Hierarchy—Cont'd**

These lower levels of need are particularly evident in health care, with the stress and anxiety of medical needs. Little progress can be made until these basic needs are met.

Self-esteem or ego needs provide us with pride of accomplishment and the respect of those we value. If all other lower needs are met, we become restless if we do not earn or feel respect. This need may be compromised if our life role and our definition of who we are changes. For example, consider the young father who no longer can support his family, or the mother who cannot care for her infant. The definition of "self" must change when we cannot fill the roles we have made for ourselves. For our patients, how they perceive the loss of esteem or ego determines its importance; for example, a small facial scar may not look disfiguring to us, but may be devastating to an actress or model. Arthritis may be manageable to most people, but if it keeps artists or pianists from practicing their skills, the esteem/ego level of need is not met.

Self-actualization is possible only if all other needs are met and we can reach our full potential. We accept ourselves and others because we are fulfilled. We can focus on outside interests with all of our needs met and can respect the opinions and beliefs of others without feeling threatened. At this level, we seek and follow medical advice and generally are our most compliant.

Remember that compliance and **adherence** imply that patients are following someone else's rules. These are, after all, "Doctor's orders." Patients may not follow preventive measures to ensure health, then may not stay with a program to correct problems brought on by the failure to follow the first directives. Patients may raise or lower medication dosages without consulting the physician; they may not complete the dosage or may not take the medication as ordered, leading to misdiagnosis when the prescribed treatment does not work. Even if patients are not responding or recovering as they should, they may not keep follow-up appointments. You may wonder, "Is he willfully disregarding his health, or did he misunderstand the importance of the health care plan?" Remember that health care is only one of life's concerns for our patients. Patients are juggling work, families, finances, and so forth, and may not see health care as the most important obligation. When the choice is between food and medicine, medicine may not be the choice. When there is time for only work and family, there may not be time for life-saving lifestyle changes, such as exercise and nutritious meals. Although as health care professionals we know that without health not much else is possible, these are hard choices to make for many of our patients.

If treatments and lifestyle changes are long-term and complicated, strict and ongoing adherence to a health care plan is less likely. Compliance is usually hard to maintain if the disorder is chronic and not particularly debilitating, such as early stages of hypertension or non–insulin-dependent diabetes mellitus, as compared to acute and painful disorders, such as a severe migraine headache. Patients follow most measures to the letter to relieve pain or nausea. However, lifestyle changes are harder to maintain over time, since results usually are not measurable on a daily basis. Many patients choose the parts of the routine that interfere least with how they prefer to live. For example, your patient's instructions are to exercise more, stop smoking, eat right, and get more rest. Some will choose to slightly modify their diet, cut down to one pack a day, and go to bed a few minutes earlier or sleep a little later.

Since the healthy changes have no immediate impact, total compliance is less likely. Conversely, if the plan quickly reverses pain or nausea, compliance is usually very high. The goal is to help patients maintain compliance for long-term changes as well as they do for short-term illnesses.

Determining the best method of strengthening compliance to patient education is a whole-team effort and will not rest on any single team member. Questions to help determine why the patient is noncompliant may include the following:

- How involved is the family, especially a spouse or parent? Compliance is far more likely if recovery becomes a joint effort, including supportive caregivers who are genuinely committed to the patient's recovery.
- Were the patient and caregiver included in the planning process? Most people are more cooperative if given choices that consider individual needs. Let those most intimately affected have a say in the learning goals and objectives.
- Have caregivers or family members lost patience with the patient? Have they found the changes and sacrifices too disruptive? Can these changes be modified to be more acceptable to the patient and caregivers?
- Is this **noncompliance**, or poor communication of information? Did the patient understand what she must do? Was the process explained appropriately? Did you use your best communication skills to ensure that she understood?
- Did he understand the importance of the directions he was given? Did he think the directions were optional?
- Do the directives go against his cultural beliefs? Does his culture believe that illness and healing are divinely ordained and beyond his control? Will his culture continue to accept him in the group if the changes he must make are deeply prohibited?
- Does she have limited resources to manage the process? These resources may include emotional, financial, supportive, or intellectual. What she was told to do may be too emotionally exhausting, too expensive, beyond her physical means, or beyond her ability to understand. In any of those situations, is it possible to adapt the patient education and health care measures to her needs?
- Finally, what is your relationship with the patient? Does he trust you? Can he tell you why he is not able to do this or why he is so resistant to compliance without fearing that you will withhold care or approval?

Patients must understand that if we do not know that directions are not being followed and if healing is not taking place, the physician may make unnecessary and possibly dangerous adjustments to the treatment. Suppose Mr. Smith is ashamed to tell you that he is not taking his antihypertensive medication as ordered because it is expensive and he is currently out of work. If he returns for evaluation and his pressure is still high, the physician may increase the dosage. If Mr. Smith then is able to take it as it is now prescribed, the dosage will be too high and may be dangerous. Most patients genuinely want to get well; if they understand the importance of following directions, they generally will comply. If they trust their health care providers, they are more likely to keep us informed of their progress.

Since it is common for compliance to gradually decline, frequent evaluations are needed to make sure that patients continue to follow healthy patterns of behavior, and that directions are followed appropriately. Patients have a right to refuse or discontinue treatment without asking for our permission, but we must try to determine why they have chosen to do this and to persuade them to return to therapies that are in their best interest.

Anytime that you feel the patient is not compliant, first check for understanding. If the patient understands the concepts and consequences but he refuses to comply, this must be documented and brought to the physician's attention.

The Hypochondriac and Playing the Sick Role

The noncompliant patient, the hypochondriac, and those who play the "sick role" are not incapable of learning and complying, but all have reasons for not following the health care plan. Our goal is to find the reasons and ensure that each patient understands why the physician's recommendations are so important.

There are almost as many advantages as disadvantages in being ill. When we are sick, we may not have to do things we would rather avoid, such as work, or participate in unpleasant social situations, or honor unwelcome obligations. However, except for the hypochondriac, most people eventually move beyond the need to escape into illness; we generally see that we must get better as our friends and families and those responsible for our care lose patience and begin to reduce the rewards of being sick.

Hypochondriacs usually have a long history of escaping into "illness behaviors." Hypochondriasis, the condition of being a hypochondriac, is also called *somatoform* or *somatic disorder* (*soma* means "body") and usually is associated with many other signs of poorly developed personality traits, such as severe anxiety, inappropriate coping skills (covered in Chapter 5, "Communicating Wellness"), and a wide range of illnesses for which there is no physical basis. They become very demanding and manipulative, and frequently tell health care workers exactly what they think their symptoms mean and are angry when no diagnostic studies or physical findings agree with their diagnosis. When the current physician cannot find a reason for the complaints, these patients frequently "doctor shop" until they find one who will agree to treat their ever-varying list of self-diagnosed illnesses. They frequently start and stop treatments as they decide which are the least intrusive, expensive, or likely to make them well. To be well means to face life without the shield of illness.

Many who play the sick role are not fully aware that this what they are doing and do not consistently demonstrate the deep-seated anxiety seen in the hypochondriac patient. Much of our behavior is family-learned, as is our response to illness and stress. These behaviors may have been formed when a child was able to escape responsibility or gather lots of rewarding attention. At the least sign of illness some children are put to bed with warm soup, a bed full of toys, and the comfort of a hovering parent. Others are told to take an aspirin and go on to school. Patients who enjoy the sick role, as opposed to the true hypochondriac, usually do well when stress is low. They truly feel ill, with vague symptoms that on examination have no consistent physical origin. For example, as a response to stress, blood pressure and heart rate may be slightly but not significantly elevated, and no physical findings support the signs. Once the need to escape has passed, sick-role patients usually return to their responsibilities until they are overwhelmed again. If we look and act sick enough, we are excused from taking part in whatever we would rather avoid. Exhibiting physical signs and symptoms of illness and seeking medical help is seen by some as more acceptable than seeking psychiatric or psychological counseling to function in stressful situations. Illness can be a very handy escape.

If the response to illness brings enough satisfaction and stress is not relieved, these patients become more manipulative, needing more health care and diagnostic tests that result in no particular new physical discoveries. They need more reassurance, and as those around them lose patience, new symptoms are created to maintain the barrier against the world.

Sick-role patients and hypochondriacs do not want to suffer. The reasons for choosing these behaviors are as individual as the patients themselves, but most truly do not want to be ill. They want the rewards they earn by being ill. It appears that what they want is the attention, care, compassion, consideration, and relief from demands that they have only when they are ill, and probably at no other time. Remember that imagined symptoms (pain, nausea, dizziness) are just as bad as symptoms with a physical origin; do not treat patients you suspect are playing these roles differently than any other patient. We have a duty to care for patients regardless of the reason for their problems. We must determine what these patients need and how we can help. If gently caring for them helps, this may be as therapeutic as any sophisticated medical treatment. Remember also that we are not trained to diagnose illness. This time the patient really may be sick; it is not up to us to decide.

How to Make Learning Easier

When the time is right and the patient is ready and motivated to learn, the process is much easier. However, we must be ready and able to teach as much as we can when the need is present. You can make a less-than-ideal learning situation easier by finding the answers to these questions and following the suggestions.

- What is the patient's favored method of learning: cognitive, affective, or psychomotor? Emphasize the preferred method, but if you incorporate all three, most patients are better able to retain and recall information.
- What does she already know about her condition? What does she need to know? And what does she want to know? If she knows almost nothing about her illness and does not want the information, she will not retain it.
- How much of the information does he need today? How much can he grasp without becoming overwhelmed? Too much information can lead to overload when the patient is already stressed. Do not burden the patient with more information than he needs to know or can comprehend at this time.
- Are you using terms familiar to the patient and appropriate for her educational level? Speak to her at her level; we need to educate, not to impress or confuse.
- Can your instructions be specific? Terms such as *small*, *large*, *pain*, and *discomfort* are subjective and vary in their interpretation.
- If you plan to reinforce today's subject with take-home information, is the material at her level of understanding? If it includes videos or audiocassettes, does she have access to the proper electronic equipment?
- If instruments and equipment are involved, did you have the patient hold and manipulate the items as you explained the purpose and use of each? Did you ask for questions at each step?
- Did you have the patient demonstrate the technique and praise him at each step as he mastered the skills? Did he understand what is expected of the treatment?
- Are group teaching sessions an option? These work well to generate support and also may result in many more questions than some patients might think to ask. Follow group teaching with one-on-one sessions at a later date.
- Did you summarize the main topics before concluding the session to make sure the patient understood?

- Did you set a time for reevaluation? This is usually done at the next scheduled visit, but you may stress to the patient to call for questions or set up a call-back schedule if you suspect he will not call you.
- Did you document the teaching and how you felt about the patient's understanding?

If it is practical and possible, provide information to take home in a form that will be understandable to the patient and have him or her review it before the scheduled information session. Tell the patient to mark areas of concern and to write questions that can be answered when you go over the material together. This will also alert you to comprehension problems. If the patient has no questions or comments, it may mean that he did not understand the information. If it is not possible to supply the material before beginning, have a copy available for the patient when the session is finished. This can be brought back at the follow-up evaluation with questions and concerns noted at that time.

Everyone responds well to positive reinforcement. As you evaluate the patient's understanding and compliance, tell him how well he is doing on those points performed or followed correctly. Most patients genuinely want to take charge of their health care. Try statements such as, "You understood (or performed) that quickly and well. Now let's go over the next point."

Measuring Literacy Levels

Physical appearance, verbal skills, and business success are not reliable indicators of literacy levels. Low literacy is the "invisible handicap," forcing people to develop other skills when they do not read or comprehend well. Many nonreaders become very good at reading visual cues and at memorizing what they see and hear to compensate for not being able to read. They become very good at manipulating others to read for them. They may offer excuses such as "I'm too sick today; read it for me," or "... too dizzy," "... too stressed," "I forgot my glasses," and so forth. Patients may promise to take the information home to read later, when you suspect they will not. Other indicators may include not reading signs posted in the facility; for example, patients may not know that payment is due at the time of service though the sign is prominently displayed in the reception area. They may look puzzled when handed reading material, or may respond inappropriately if they misunderstand what most people could read easily. We must never embarrass our patients by pointing out a deficiency of any sort, and most particularly one so potentially devastating to self-esteem. However, we must, at least initially, determine whether patients can read well enough to follow written instructions that they do not see in everyday situations, such as "Stop," "Go," "Ladies," "Gentlemen," etc. Common instructions and directions such as those are mastered by sight by most nonreaders. We will cover more complex methods of determining reading levels below, but assessment tools are not always practical in a hurried situation. These simple steps will suggest a patient's low literacy skills.

- Give him something to read, for example a brochure or information regarding his diagnosis.
- Ask him questions about what he read and what he thought about it.

If he stammers about for an answer, suspect that he cannot read or comprehend at a level to understand medical information. Remember, for legal as well as ethical purposes, instructions must be understood for informed consent. Patients must understand, and many with low literacy levels cannot.

Patients with learning disabilities have a neurological dysfunction that prevents them from mastering a certain skill, such as reading, writing, or other method of communicating that disrupts the ability to learn. Many younger patients have learning disabilities diagnosed early in their school years and are given the help they need for lifelong learning. However, many still slip through the educational cracks, and others who are older were never diagnosed in time to overcome this barrier to learning. It is not in our scope of practice to educate patients to read and comprehend; however, it is our responsibility to ensure that anyone who needs our help is offered assistance at a level to benefit his or her health status, and in some cases that will mean assisting with reading comprehension.

Low literacy, for those who are not learning disabled, is defined by most sources as reading at a 5th to 8th grade level. These persons may read, write, and comprehend but at a level far below the skills needed to understand most medical information, which generally is written at a high school or higher level. Others may have difficulty comprehending both spoken and written language beyond a certain level of complexity. They may understand instructions both written and spoken at a grade-school level, but are confused at anything presented in a higher level format. Unfortunately, graduating from high school does not necessarily indicate 12th-grade reading skills, since many graduates read several years below their grade level.

Many people with low literacy levels are considered functionally illiterate with a limited ability to comprehend or communicate by written or spoken language. They may read the words correctly and may hear what you say but will not understand the context or meaning. The functionally illiterate patient probably will return for health care frequently because he is not able to follow instructions for restoring or maintaining health. Low literacy is a large factor in poor health and high medical costs; these patients do not have the literacy skills needed to learn to care for themselves.

It is not practical in many situations to evaluate reading skills for patients in our busy medical facilities, but evaluation methods are available to determine literacy levels when it is vital to provide information at an understandable level. Medical facilities responsible for educating patients for long-term lifestyle changes or chronic disease management need to know their patients' reading levels to design education material appropriate for individual patients. Box 4-2 covers methods of determining reading levels when it is important that patients read and understand printed directives for at-home care.

Box **4-2**   **Evaluating Literacy Levels**

Two recognized methods of evaluating reading levels include the Wide Range Achievement Test (WRAT) and the Rapid Estimate of Adult Literacy in Medicine (REALM). WRAT has the reader recognize and pronounce words on a test that should take about 5 minutes. There are two testing levels, one for children ages 5 through 12, and one for persons older than 12 years. REALM assesses how well the reader understands medical concepts rather than simply reading levels. The patient reads aloud from three lists of medical words from simple to complex. The total number of words the patient can read gives the score. Both tests require that the patient read the words but may not evaluate whether or not the patient understands what he is reading. Some patients can read but cannot tell you what the sentence means. The Cloze Test evaluates reading levels above the 6th-grade level and tests for understanding as well as word recognition. Comprehension is measured by having the patient read short sections of the test with blanks where certain words should be. Those taking the test must understand the content of the text to supply the missing words.

After determining the patient's reading level, match it to patient education material (PEM) designed for the appropriate level. Most material can be restructured from high literacy levels to lower levels without losing effectiveness. In fact, material written at a level beyond the patient's grasp cannot be considered effective. The level at which printed material is written can be evaluated by several software scanning systems. They generally scan several pages and compare the length of words, sentences, and paragraphs to various proposed grade levels. Examples include the Flesch Test, which evaluates grades 5 through college, the Fog test for grades 4 through college, and the Fry test for grades 1 through college. Other tools are in development or already in use, but all use the same concept. If your facility has found that reading levels and comprehension in your population is a concern, these programs can enhance your written communication and increase patient compliance, which is the goal of all patient education and communication.

Working with Caregivers

This chapter has concentrated on educating patients in self-care. In many cases, however, it is necessary or more appropriate to educate caregivers. Examples include parents of young children, guardians of developmentally deficient persons of any age, or caregivers of elderly patients with dementia. Also, as mentioned earlier, some cultures require that women act as caregivers, in which case, the men of the group may refuse to listen to instructions that will be assigned to the women of the group. Determine who will be administering care and include that person or persons in the education sessions.

We have talked of determining the patient's readiness and ability to learn, but the caregiver should be assessed also, particularly if most of the care will fall on one caregiver, rather than being shared by the patient, other family members, or outside agencies, such as home health or a visiting nurse. Caregivers who are not capable of caring for a very sick person will soon be sick themselves, and your patient will be no better. Determine whether the caregiver is physically, mentally, emotionally, and financially able to care for the patient at the level the patient requires and if the caregiver is motivated to care for the patient. All of the points we have considered in determining readiness and comprehension apply to both patient and caregiver and should be evaluated and documented.

In any of the above situations, or others that you might encounter, all of the teaching factors described in this chapter apply. As much as possible, include the patient, but if his condition prevents comprehension or compliance, you must concentrate on educating those responsible for his care and incorporating their needs as well as the patient's into the educational material.

Working with Children

As noted in discussing barriers to communicating with children, the range of ages and developmental abilities in children present challenges not usually encountered with adults. This does not mean that we should not make every effort to talk with children, even young ones, about how to live a healthy lifestyle. Many adult illnesses have their roots in childhood habits and can be prevented if children understand at an age-appropriate level the importance of healthy living with diet and exercise. Children also have a number of illnesses that require at least partial self-management that we may have to teach. These include the rising rates of asthma requiring inhalers and spirometer readings, juvenile-onset diabetes requiring glucose testing and insulin, and many congenital anomalies (birth defects) and disorders that require treatment and management.

Responsible adults and caregivers must be present for education sessions, especially with young children. They need to understand how much the child can and should do alone, but children almost always need someone to supervise compliance and to ensure that procedures are performed correctly. As the child matures in the illness, supervision may become less intrusive but still should be available at regular intervals.

To communicate with children during the education process, review our earlier suggestions for overcoming communication barriers, particularly those for children, and try these methods:

- Build trust with the child by being honest, and do not betray that trust. If it will hurt, tell her so.
- Limit sessions to no more than 10 minutes. If the child's attention span is particularly short, even 10 minutes may be too long.
- Use dolls and the proper equipment. Let children handle and touch the tools they will use to manage their illness.
- Use age-appropriate language and explanations. Do not expect a 5-year-old to understand the same concepts available to a 10-year-old.
- Praise, praise, praise. We all enjoy being told we have done a good job; watch children glow at your praise.
- If appropriate, include in the planning the question, "Can you do this?" If the skill is too difficult, frightening, or upsetting, the child may not be ready.
- Use age-appropriate coloring books and booklets to help explain difficult concepts.
- Expect regression during an illness. A 6-year-old may act like a 4-year-old when he is ill. This is normal. Do not ridicule the child or try to shame him into mature behavior.
- Give children as much information as they need, but do not overwhelm them with concepts they do not need at this time.
- Adolescents resent authority, fear loss of body image or being different, and will be very upset at having to return to a former level of dependence just as they are reaching for autonomy. Expect anger and resistance and use tact and diplomacy.
- Teenagers may seem mature enough to understand but may not relate to preventive measures, such as, "If you do this now, you will have fewer problems later." Because many presume they will never grow older, they may not listen; if you suspect this is true, focus on the immediate needs at this time. However, never miss a chance to stress a prudent lifestyle, since some of the information may register for future reference.

The Importance of Support Groups

Even in North America with our strongly independent character, we still need support from those who care about us. Remember Maslow's "love and belonging" level of social needs? Remember, too, that this level closely follows safety and security. If we have no support group, we have no safety net; we do not belong. As independent as we claim to be, we still need help much of the time, especially when we are sick.

Many studies show that patients with a strong support group are more likely to recover. People in good, supportive relationships, whether married or not, are healthier than those who are widowed, divorced, or who have no significant other. We all need support from family, our social group, or a group with similar interests and goals. This seems to be a strong, basic human need and is vital to recovery from illness. If patients know that someone or something loves and depends on them, they usually make every effort to comply with education and instructions so that they can hurry home. Consider the mother of young children versus an elderly, childless widower. Who do you think will make the greatest effort to recover quickly? Even if the loved one waiting is a pet, not a person, patients will do everything necessary to return home if they know someone needs them. Going home to loneliness may delay recovery.

The groups to which we belong for support include the following:

A *family*, in any sense of the word, implies a mutually supportive relationship. The concept of traditional, or nuclear, families with two opposite-sex parents and 2.5 children has evolved to mean many arrangements and assortments. The term *family* now loosely means a group of people living together or closely connected by bonds of interdependence. The members have common concerns and meet each other's needs for safety, security, love, and belonging. Illness for one affects the whole group.

Families are affected differently depending on the age of the patient and the extent of the illness. If the family is close and loving, everyone is affected by the illness of any one of its members, but if the patient is elderly and incapacitated versus a young child or a vital young parent, the response may be different. How the family reacts depends on how severely the illness affects the family dynamics. A sick child is devastating to the whole family and makes immense demands on the parents and other siblings. A sick parent cannot productively contribute to the family safety and security and is a source of anxiety rather than comfort. An elderly relative may be loved unconditionally, but if the illness is long and debilitating, the family unit may learn to work around the illness more easily than for a more productive member of the family.

Working with a family in health care may require interaction with more than one caregiver or family member. Many viewpoints may have to be coordinated. For example, consider an elderly, dependent grandparent: one family member may feel that long-term care is more appropriate than home care, whereas another may feel that long-term care is a last resort. Some members may want a "do not resuscitate" (DNR) order signed, whereas others may strongly resist. All of these areas of family care require great tact and understanding. These families usually are dealing with the same need for emotional support as the patient and have no emotional resources left for themselves or the patient. Any illness causes great stress to the whole family unit.

Structured *support groups* are fairly formal, with leaders, time frames for meetings, tasks to perform, and roles for the members. These roles include those who need information and those who provide it, those who offer support and those who seek it. A facilitator usually helps motivate the group, keeps it together, keeps it on task, and assigns and coordinates the regularly scheduled meetings. Facilitators help avoid group dysfunction, such as aggression, dominating personalities, and critics. Examples of structured support groups are Alcoholics Anonymous, Reach for Recovery (post-mastectomy), Candlelighters (parents of children with cancer), and groups coordinated by associations such as The Muscular Dystrophy Association, The National Kidney Foundation, and so forth. There is a support group for most common illnesses.

Many patients join these groups and find that helping others helps them deal with their own illness (Fig. 4-2). If patients can see how others are adjusting and how they handle the illness, their own hopelessness and helplessness are relieved. Members usually are in varying stages of successful coping and can help with the best ways to approach complications, access resources, and so on. Seeing others who are doing well makes changes less stressful, and if

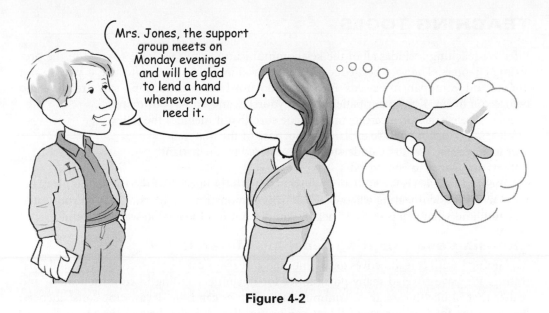

Figure 4-2

one member is not doing well, others gain strength by offering support. Since many of the patient's social supports, such as work, sports, or school, are no longer as available as before the illness, or the members of previous social groups are not as understanding and supportive, the new support group will be illness-based. This may be what the patient and his caregivers need at this time. This new concentration on the illness may interfere with a well-rounded life, but as the illness is incorporated into a new lifestyle, former social supports, such as friends and coworkers, may be resumed, and less emphasis can be placed on the formal support group.

Research the support groups in your area to be certain the philosophies of the group agree with the physician's manner of treating the illness. If the physician's directions and the group's suggestions are opposed, the patient and caregivers will be understandably stressed and confused.

Social groups are loosely woven and less formal than families or structured support groups. These include neighbors, religious groups, and groups of friends. The members may care for each other at least as well as some families. They check on each other, run errands, coordinate meals, and fill many needs. These groups may lack commitment, but any successful social support group usually has someone who keeps things going by coordinating the efforts of the others.

Interdependent or collective cultures usually have better support than some areas of North American culture. If collective cultures move away from extended family, they tend to settle into communities with like-minded neighbors who become their family in time of need. Most Americans value independence of thought and lifestyle, and many tend to move from areas with strong ties to places with only fragile links to the local community. Americans frequently are scattered, and even **estranged**, from family and friends. This loss of the safety/security and love/belonging hierarchical needs adds to the stress of illness.

TEACHING TOOLS

Effective teaching includes all of the key communication skills we have covered in the preceding chapters. The very best educational material available is less effective if you do not understand your patient's needs and if you do not have a good, supportive relationship before you begin. Know your patient, know yourself, and know your material.

As you select, adapt, or create material, be sure that it includes the following:
- A learning goal or goals to explain the purpose of the material
- Learning objectives to be understood or mastered by the patient
- Items and issues to be covered
- A method or criteria for evaluating the outcome or the success of the education process
- An area for documenting whether the patient demonstrated understanding to your satisfaction and what you plan to do next if you did not feel the session was successful

Choosing and Adapting Teaching Material

Explaining health care directives to patients and caregivers can be time-consuming and frustrating. We have covered many possibilities for misunderstanding in communication and realize that in health care, these communication lapses can have devastating consequences. Because time for teaching may fall between hectic clinical duties, having commercially prepared patient education material (PEM) at hand can be a great time-saver. For example, most orthopedists have user-friendly guides for cast care and crutch walking in booklet form, and many also have the PEM in video form. After explaining and demonstrating cast care guidelines and crutch safety, for example, having appropriate PEM streamlines the procedure and more likely ensures that patients will remember or can refer to key points at home. These types of PEM usually are available in various levels of reading or learning styles, contain brightly colored and appealing illustrations, and include accepted medical practice. When choosing an assortment of materials, it is better to have a few well-written resources than many that cover the material inadequately.

Prepackaged education materials are also available as computer programs that allow the user to individualize the material to specific situations. They usually present a variety of formats, such as a suggested outline to fill in with the doctor's preference for this patient, or a more complete plan that needs only minor additions or adaptations. These make better use of your time than creating what is already professionally available. They make it easy to adapt the information for the physician and patient. These resources are available for patients with different communication needs also, such as the patient who speaks English as a second language or has impairments such as vision deficits.

If your patient is comfortable with a computer, several reputable sites have very good information for patients to access from home. Some sites offer interactive patient education for reinforcement and patient participation in learning. Be sure that the physician approves of the sites used as reference before recommending them to patients.

Patient education material has been created by most of the organized groups supporting various illnesses, such as the many brochures, booklets, and audiovisual aids provided for diabetes or cancer support, hypertension, heart disease, and gastrointestinal disorders. For example, the American Heart Association and the American Cancer Society have very good PEM. This material is well written at many levels but may not be specific enough for each patient's needs or to fit each physician's philosophy. Before presenting proposed information to the physician for consideration, think about your patient population. Look at the overall

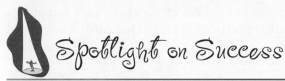

Spotlight on Success

Publicity about new health concerns can be frightening and confusing to the general public. News programs and other forms of media can create panic very quickly. For example, not long ago, many people panicked when anthrax was found in several pieces of mail. Severe acute respiratory syndrome (SARS) was a frightening epidemic even though very few people died of the disease. When these types of health issues occur, your patients will turn to you for reassurance and clarification. Listen to the nightly news or read the daily newspapers and other news journals and develop a keen interest in health-related information. Check the Internet for credible resources for your patients. Print articles and Internet sites for patients to access information for themselves. Taking the initiative to stay abreast of current trends shows your supervisor that you have the qualities looked for in a health care professional.

visual appeal, the format, the illustrations, and the vocabulary level of the material. Do you need Spanish or Vietnamese language aids? What about large print for the vision-impaired patient? Are the majority of your patients poorly educated with low reading skills, or is your facility more likely to attract highly educated patients? When you have determined what your facility needs, go over the material with the physician. Make sure it is written to comply with his or her philosophy of health care. With your close and intense personal contact, you may be more familiar with the general level of needs to determine which format would be most appropriate for your patients (see Spotlight on Success box).

Developing Teaching Material

Adapting available material and developing your own tools may use many of the same resources. Many medically oriented publishing companies provide teaching plan resource books and software programs that guide the user to an accepted teaching format. Hospital libraries usually have these formats available as hard copy or as computer programs. If you are responsible for creating or developing material for your agency, you may also find resources at local bookstores.

If no preprinted material covers medical information in a manner that your physician approves, you may prepare your own using the following guidelines:

- Decide what your patient needs to know or do and outline a desired or expected outcome.
- Keep it simple and to-the-point.
- Follow a logical order and organize from simple to complex concepts.
- Either define technical terms or reword to eliminate phrases that patients may not understand. Our object is to educate, not to impress.
- Use bold headings to prepare the reader for the upcoming topic.
- Use short sentences of no more than eight to 10 words and short paragraphs, rather than large blocks of text. The first sentence of each paragraph should alert the reader to the topic and each paragraph should cover only one topic.
- Outlines work well for patients with short attention spans.
- Highlight or bold central concepts to call attention to their importance.
- Format with wide margins to avoid overwhelming the reader.

- Use a good design layout that includes illustrations; even clip art from your computer's bank or simple diagrams help relieve blocks of text. Many readers are visual learners and need text broken up by pictured examples.
- Use a simple typeface or font. Avoid using italics, script, or unusual lettering. These are confusing to low-literacy readers.
- Use at least 12-point type. Use even larger type for older patients or those with vision impairments.
- Use good paper with good contrast. Colored paper may make it harder for some patients to read.
- Personalize the text with "you" and "your" as much as possible, rather than using an impersonal format.
- Prepare several levels of material, such as wording at a 5th-grade level and another at high school or college level. Do not confuse the low-literacy patient, and do not write below the level of the literate patient.
- After using material for a while, review it to see if it is still relevant and effective. Medical information changes quickly and should be updated as needed.

Remember that PEM is not designed to take the place of interacting with the patient; it is a teaching aid, not a substitute.

When you are confident that your patient and his caregiver understand the health care concerns and that each is competent to continue home care and adopt a prudent lifestyle, you will have given them the independence that is the goal of quality health care.

 Taking the Chapter to Work

Now, let's meet Jacob and Francine and see how they have applied this chapter information in the workplace.

Jacob is working in a community clinic setting. He is interviewing a 42-year-old man who has experienced the following changes in the past three months: divorce, job loss, and filed for bankruptcy. The patient has come to the clinic because last night he tripped and fell on a curb at 2 a.m. and is complaining of ankle pain. Jacob asks the patient if he had ingested any alcoholic beverages prior to the fall. The patient begins crying and states that he has a few drinks every night to help "cope" with life's stresses. Jacob offers the patient some brochures about alcoholism and provides him with a schedule of the local Alcoholics Anonymous support groups. Jacob communicates this information to the physician. Although the purpose of the visit was the ankle injury, Jacob's questioning was able to identify a problem that needed intervention and he utilized available resources.

Francine is working in a surgeon's office. She is caring for a patient who has multiple ulcers on her lower extremities. After the surgeon examined the patient, he asked Francine to apply gauze and compression stockings to the patient's legs. Francine used this opportunity to teach psychomotor skills. She explained why the dressings were important and then demonstrated how to apply them. She applied the dressing to the left leg and then had the patient apply the dressing to the right leg. While the patient applied the dressing, Francine was able to provide helpful hints and suggestions. At the end of the teaching session, Francine asked the patient questions to ensure comprehension.

Beyond the Classroom Exercises

Your Assignment Board

The following exercises will help you use your new knowledge. Place a check beside the assignments your instructor has given you. When you have completed the assignment, place a check in the completed column.

		Assigned	*Completed*
Checking Your Comprehension	(Textbook)	☐	☐
Expanding Critical Thinking	(Textbook)	☐	☐
Communication Surfer Exercises	(Textbook and Internet)	☐	☐
Communication Tree Branch #5	(CD-ROM)	☐	☐
Communication Tree Branch #6	(CD-ROM)	☐	☐
Voice Mail Message #4	(CD-ROM)	☐	☐
Patient/Caregiver Interview #3	(CD-ROM)	☐	☐
Patient/Caregiver Interview #4	(CD-ROM)	☐	☐

 ## Checking Your Comprehension

Write a brief answer for each of the following assignments.
1. Identify the five patient education steps. Write a short explanation of each step.
2. Describe the three basic learning styles.
3. Give examples of the five most common implementation methods. Write a short explanation of each method.
4. Describe four factors that can make learning harder. Prepare a list of actions you can take to help overcome these factors.
5. Name the five steps of Maslow's hierarchy of needs and explain how illness may affect each level.
6. Write six questions that you can ask to determine whether the patient is noncompliant.
7. Summarize the responsibilities of a support group facilitator.

Expanding Critical Thinking

1. Demonstrate to another student how to wrap an elastic bandage as if the student does not understand English well. Explain how to obtain a clean-catch, midstream urine specimen. Explain range of motion (ROM) exercises or crutch-walking. Have the student evaluate how well you explained each situation. Now change roles.
2. List some of the gains associated with the sick role. Give examples of the obligations that might be avoided by adopting the sick role.
3. Which of the barriers to communication covered in Chapter 2 do you think would make patient education most difficult? Describe ways to overcome the following barriers in a teaching situation:
   a. Explain insulin self-injection to a 70-year-old man with progressive vision loss.
   b. Teach crutch gaits to a 40-year-old woman with a hearing impairment.

Continued

Expanding Critical Thinking—Cont'd

    c. Describe collecting a urine specimen to a 65-year-old post-CVA (cerebrovascular accident) man with a cognitive language impairment.

    d. Explain how to collect a stool specimen for occult blood to a 35-year-old father who thinks he has colon cancer.

    e. Describe an appropriate diet to a 6-year-old child with juvenile diabetes.

    f. Stress the importance of prudent diet choices to an overweight teenager with early-stage hypertension.

    g. Explain home safety measure to a 90-year-old who has begun to fall frequently.

4. Look back at Maslow's Hierarchy of Needs. Where do you think the following people are on the pyramid: A young mother in a war-torn country; an artist at a showing of her award-winning sculpture; a young man in the initiation ritual into a gang in a dangerous inner city; a young husband working his way up the corporate ladder. Is the communication level different among these people? If so, how? Which person would you feel the most comfortable communicating with? With whom would you feel least comfortable and why?

5. List three situations that may make you uncomfortable teaching patients. Would you be more comfortable if the patient were about your same age and your same sex? How would you feel if the patient is older than you? Younger than you? The opposite sex? How could you overcome your discomfort in each situation?

6. Mr. Carter is 85 and has recently suffered a CVA and will need assistance at home with activities of daily living (ADLs), such as toiletting, bathing, dressing and eating, as well as ROM exercises to increase his mobility. Mrs. Carter is his only relative and is a frail 83-year-old. In your opinion, do you think she is capable of his unassisted care? What should you do to help her to ensure that both patient and caregiver benefit during his recuperation? How would you communicate this need?

 Communication Surfer Exercises

1. Choose three diseases that you would like to learn more information about. Now, using the Internet, find a site for each of these diseases that would help patients better understand their illnesses.

2. You need to teach a patient a new skill but the patient does not speak English. Find three Internet sites that would be help you communicate or could provide resources to help with this patient.

3. A caregiver of an elderly parent verbalizes the need for help and support. Find five Internet sites that help caregivers manage the daily struggles of caring for a sick person at home.

4. Using a search engine, type in the word "education." How many results did you get? What terms could you use to narrow your search to find sites that help you develop or find patient education materials?

5. Support groups can often be very helpful for a patient. Using the Internet, find at least 20 different types of support groups. Visit all 20 sites. Then make a list of the 10 best sites. What made these sites good? What did you find helpful about these sites?

5

COMMUNICATING WELLNESS: WHAT DOES IT TAKE TO BE HEALTHY?

LEARNING OBJECTIVES

Upon successfully completing this chapter, you will be able to:

- State the factors that help determine our health status.
- Assist in planning and explaining a diet appropriate for a variety of medical needs.
- Explain how to adjust dietary needs for ethnic and age diversity.
- Differentiate between food-related medical disorders.
- List various exercise options and explain the benefits of each.
- Differentiate between positive and negative stress and give the physiologic effects of each.
- Describe ways to incorporate relaxation and stress relief techniques into patient education.
- Compare methods of coping with stress and determine which are appropriate in various medically related situations.
- State ways to recognize suicidal potential and list means of helping patients avoid this option.
- Identify substances that commonly lead to abuse and addiction, and describe their effects on the body.
- List information to include in educating patients about medication therapy.
- Describe ways to ensure the physical safety of various age groups.
- Give examples of incorporating alternative and/or complementary medicine into traditional medical therapy.

KEY TERMS

Bariatric	Exchanges	Negative stress
Catatonic	Exercise	Organic
Coping	Exogenous	Positive stress
Endogenous	Invincibility	Range of motion
Euphoria	Maladaptive	
Eustress	Manic	

Test Your Communication IQ

Before reading this chapter, complete this short self-assessment test. Decide which statements are true and which are false.

1. To achieve wellness, you must focus on prevention rather than "fixing" the problem.
2. When talking with patients about fad diets, it is important to communicate that two people consuming the same diet often will have different results because they metabolize their food differently.
3. It is important to communicate to vegetarians that this diet cannot meet their nutritional needs.
4. It is important to communicate that exercise can decrease immune cell production and can lower cholesterol levels.
5. The parasympathetic nervous system works to calm the body's reaction to stress.
6. It is important to communicate to patients how stress affects the body.
7. Suicide rates decrease during holiday times.
8. When communicating with patients who are addicted, increasing their feelings of guilt will promote recovery.

Results

Statements three, four, seven, and eight are false; all others are true. How did you do? Read the chapter to find more information on these topics.

In this technological age, "experts" bombard us with information to make us better looking, more intelligent, and more muscular, to grow more hair, and to lose weight overnight. Since all of this is certainly too good to be true, patients rely on health care providers to know and understand the best means of maintaining or restoring health. Therefore, we must understand the basis of a healthy lifestyle to help patients sort through media information and misinformation. Since many educational opportunities are spur-of-the-moment, we need a firm knowledge of prudent living to answer promptly and correctly when patients ask about the latest "infomercial" or Internet miracle.

The health care profession understands that no matter how advanced technology becomes in correcting illnesses, prevention is still the best defense. By understanding how certain factors influence health, either for better or for worse, and how to incorporate healthy choices in lifestyle behaviors, we can help educate patients to work toward achieving or maintaining the best possible level of health. It is not the purpose of this text to teach or explain the physiology of the human body. For example, anatomy and physiology or human biology courses cover how the body works to absorb and metabolize nutrients, how it works through exercise to build strong muscles and bones, and how it coordinates the stress response by secreting enzymes that prepare us to battle stress. Our goal is to help you communicate what you learn in science courses in a manner that patients can understand. Combining the knowledge earned in other courses with a comfortable, communicative rapport with your patients helps you transmit the information needed to restore or maintain health. The range of potential teaching topics is extensive and varies with the patient, the illness, and the specialty. The topics we selected to discuss here are those that health care professionals address most frequently. These include teaching patients about nutrition, exercise, stress, substance abuse, medication therapy, safety, and alternatives to traditional medicine.

WHAT MAKES US SICK

Wellness is not simply an absence of disease; wellness is attaining the best health status possible regardless of existing physical conditions. Patients with heart disease or diabetes mellitus, both life-changing and life-threatening diseases, can achieve maximum wellness within the limits of these diseases. Likewise, a patient with a physical disability may consider himself healthy, while an otherwise healthy person with an acute illness, such as an influenza virus, may consider himself sick. For example, Mrs. Smith has insulin-dependent diabetes mellitus and hypertension, both of which affect her quality of life but both are currently under control. If you ask her how she feels today, she may answer that she is doing well. On the other hand, Joe Brown is in excellent health, but has the latest 24-hour gastrointestinal virus and feels terrible. He will tell you quickly how very sick he is. The feeling of wellness in both cases is relative to the patient's normal state of health.

Somewhere between premature death and glowing good health is a state of wellness acceptable to most people trying to maintain a healthy balance. We would like to think that every patient will work toward being as healthy as individually possible, but some will accept a lower level of fitness if achieving good health means giving up cherished lifestyle behaviors such as cigarettes or high-fat fast food. One of our main responsibilities lies in convincing patients that wellness is a goal worth pursuing.

Achieving wellness works best by prevention, rather than "fixing" something that is not working. We must help patients understand that it is better to work to maintain good health than to correct preventable diseases and disorders such as elevated blood pressure or increased levels of cholesterol after they are established. Heart disease, liver disease, certain types of ulcers, HIV and sexually transmitted diseases (STDs), and many types of cancer can be brought on by our own behavior. Prevention begins long before symptoms appear and patients turn to us for help.

One of our goals as health care professionals is to educate patients in the holistic approach to health. All factors of our "self" must come together for the self-actualization level that includes wellness (refer to Chapter 4, "Educating Patients," for Maslow's Hierarchy of Needs). Holistic medicine works for harmony and balance, or homeostasis, in all areas that make us who we are (Fig. 5-1). This includes our physical being, our mental or emotional self, and our social life and spirituality. Patients are ultimately responsible for maintaining this balance, we cannot do it for them, but we must help them learn to maintain wellness using natural means and prudent choices before they need medical intervention.

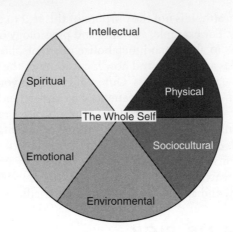

Figure 5-1
Circle of Life: The "whole" of a person is greater than and different from the sum of the parts.

Through all of our discussions of health, remember that disease is only one of the many parts of the person we are treating; we must consider the whole person. Medical science has always linked healthy minds to healthy bodies. Illness was originally thought to be evil spirits invading the mind and directing the body. Now we have scientific evidence that a healthy mind nurtures a healthy body and vice versa. Our mind and our body make up our total self; if the health of one is affected, it may be devastating to the whole self. The whole patient includes the following:
- Physical health and fitness
- Mental health and emotional stability
- Stress management
- Environmental and occupational safety
- Social supports
- Spiritual harmony
  Many factors work together for holistic health. They include the following:
- *Genetic endowment*: Along with general appearance and other characteristics, we inherit our anatomy and physiology, metabolism, and immune system from our extended family. For example, how well our body resists communicable diseases depends on a strong and intact immune system. Some people never seem to catch a cold or flu, and others seem to attract every passing microorganism. Preventive measures (immunizations, Standard Precautions, and so forth) are a big factor, but so is the strength of our inherited immune system. Likewise, how we metabolize dietary fats, for example, has a strong relationship to whether or not we develop heart disease. How strong and well made our body is (anatomy) and how well it works (physiology) helps determine our general level of health and resistance to disease.
- *Availability of health care (socioeconomic status)*: The world's best medical technology will not help our patients if it is not available to them. Whether a patient can afford prevention measures or to seek help to relieve a medical problem depends largely on financial resources. When the decision is between food or shelter and health care, and the question

is "Of all I must pay, which is most important?", health care, particularly preventive care, may be a low priority. Wealthy patients with better education and better access to health care usually know the symptoms of illness, have regular physical examinations, and schedule diagnostic screenings to manage illness while it is still more likely curable. Financially stable patients usually maintain immunizations for childhood diseases, flu, pneumonia, tetanus, and hepatitis B. Many poorer patients with no access to health care do not have these options.

- *Family dynamics:* A calm, loving home protects us from many stresses and meets our love/belonging and safety/security hierarchical needs. A stormy, upsetting home life gives us no shelter from the stress of the outside world. Family exposure also teaches us how to respond to illness, forms our exercise and diet habits, and shows us how to react to stress.
- *Culture*: The food we eat, our reproductive philosophies, and how we care for our illnesses are all largely cultural and have an enormous impact on health. We have covered cultural factors in the health care setting, and as we work through this text we will see how diet and cultural approaches to health care affect long-term health.
- *Environmental*: Exposure to polluted air, water, soil, or foods stresses even the strongest immune system. Environmental exposure to strong, drug-resistant microorganisms challenges our resistance and may overpower otherwise good health.
- *Emotional or physical stress*: Extremely stressful situations or exposure to moderate stress over a long period measurably decreases the immune response and makes us susceptible to opportunistic disease. This is covered later in this chapter in "The Stress Factor."
- *Poor social habits*: Smoking, alcohol and drug abuse, a sedentary lifestyle, and overexposure to sun versus good nutrition, exercise, and prudent living all strongly influence long-term health. Imprudent choices lead to STDs, traumatic injuries, early degenerative disease, and generally poor health, regardless of a strong inherited immune system.

Help-seeking mechanisms vary also and significantly affect health. Whether we seek help is very cultural and also varies with age, social class, and sex. Patients must recognize that something is wrong, realize that help is needed, and decide on a course of action. Many patients deny they have a problem if they have more pressing hierarchical needs (review Chapter 4, "Educating Patients," for Maslow's Hierarchy of Needs).

- Middle-aged and older adults ask for help more frequently than teenagers and young adults.
- Educated patients with better financial resources are more likely to recognize when they need care than members of lower socioeconomic groups with less education.
- Women ask for help more frequently than men, and mothers of young children are most likely of all to seek help.
- The patient's perception of the illness is also a factor. He may wonder, "Is this a heart attack or indigestion?" Many do not recognize a problem unless the symptoms are identifiable or unusually uncomfortable or painful. Many wait with vague symptoms before asking for help.
- If the suspected disorder or symptom is not socially acceptable, patients may decide not to seek help. Patients may wonder, "Do I want anyone to know about this?" Many patients would rather not report symptoms that are potentially embarrassing. For example, consider the following for social acceptance: a vaginal discharge that may be a STD versus a breast lump; skin cancer versus possible Kaposi's sarcoma; heart disease versus morbid obesity. Pride is associated with some disorders, such as those related to sports; for example, shin splints and tennis elbow. Patients are rarely reluctant to report these disorders.

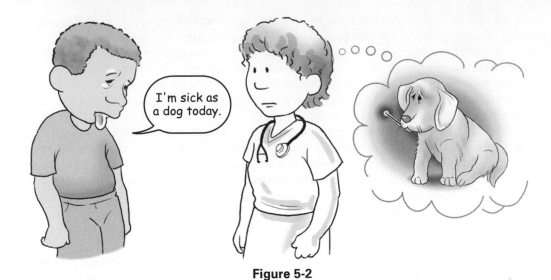

Figure 5-2

- The age at which the symptoms appear may determine whether the patient or caregiver sees the symptom or sign as significant. For example, for whom would unexplained joint pain be a greater concern, an otherwise healthy 10-year-old or an 85-year-old with multiple health problems?
- For working adults, seeking help may depend on balancing available sick leave against the severity of the symptoms. Patients may weigh the options of treating themselves or going for help if they have no more sick days available.
- The day of week and the time of day also have an impact on reporting illnesses. Patients are more likely to seek help early in the week or early in the day and are least likely to report illness on Friday or the weekend or late in the evening (Fig. 5-2). Think of what this might mean for someone with unexplained chest pain.

All of the factors listed above help determine whether patients are likely to be ill and whether they ask for help with health care problems. If they do not come to us, we cannot offer our care. Once they recognize the need, we can begin to do those things for which we were trained.

THE NUTRITION GOAL: WE ARE WHAT WE EAT

The body needs fuel from a well-balanced diet to remain healthy, delay degenerative disorders, and resist communicable illnesses. This concept is so important that many health care agencies employ nutritionists and dietitians to help patients determine a diet to meet individual needs. This is particularly important for patients with severe nutritional disorders, or with disorders caused by poor eating habits. If there are no diet specialists on staff, referrals can be made to outside sources. If the problem is not complicated or does not require close professional management, patient education materials can be ordered or created to help instruct patients regarding a healthy diet.

Diet is one of the most important of the controllable factors influencing health. The term *diet* comes from the Greek word, meaning *diata*, "a way of life." What and how we eat have such a profound affect on health that the importance of diet-related wellness throughout our lifetime cannot be overemphasized. Salt, fat, sugar, caffeine, and alcohol all significantly affect how well the body functions. Although hunger is certainly present in our country, most Americans are rarely truly hungry. However, many who can afford to eat well are obese, nutritionally deficient, or malnourished by poor diet choices; in fact, many of our most obese patients are technically malnourished. Diet-related heart disease, osteoporosis, cirrhosis, and eating disorders are more common in the United States than in most other developed nations in spite of the abundance of food, nutritional education in schools, and the constant exposure to diet theories. Patients need to know and understand the basics of good nutrition. It is human nature to eat only what we have always eaten or only what we like, unless we understand how important it is to our overall health and quality of life to vary our diet and to eat nutritious foods properly prepared.

Review your course work that includes the mechanics of metabolism and nutrition to refresh your memory of how the body uses nutrients to grow and heal. Remember these concepts as you help patients understand the importance of an appropriate diet and as you help the physician determine the patient's nutritional status. Your clinical responsibilities may include many of the measurements used to assess a patient's nutritional status. Height versus weight, fat to muscle ratio, and body mass index comparisons are reliable indicators of healthy food choices. A tool called a caliper measures skin fold thickness at various points on the body to determine subcutaneous (under the skin) fat deposits. Biochemical blood tests register levels of available nutrients in circulation. The nutritional history is also assessed in the physical examination with the physician's inspection of the patient's skin, hair, eyes, teeth, and muscle mass. To complete the analysis, a diet history helps determine how much patients understand about nutrition.

When all of the information listed above regarding the patient's nutritional status is documented and evaluated, education and an appropriate diet can be arranged around the patient's specific needs. Not everyone responds equally to the same procedures or medication, and the same is true of diets. Two people consuming the same diet respond according to their individual metabolism. One may lose significant weight; the other may simply maintain, neither gaining nor losing. If the health concern involves a nutritional imbalance, such as poor absorption of nutrients or the need for great weight loss, a dietitian or nutritionist should work with the patient. These situations will not respond to the latest best selling one-size-fits-all diet. In cases of morbid obesity, patients may be referred to a **bariatrics** specialist, a new field that concentrates on obesity and its related disorders. However, in cases that involve nothing more than poor or imprudent food choices, following the current accepted nutritional guidelines almost always leads to better health and more realistic weight regulation. Since the nutritional and dietary sciences constantly update recommendations to reflect new information regarding proper food choices, it is in everyone's best interest to stay current of the latest dietary theories. Guidelines have been designed to ensure healthy food choices for most age groups, many cultural and ethnic backgrounds, and various diseases and disorders. All can be easily adapted for individual preferences and special needs (Box 5-1).

Food Guide Pyramids

In 2005, the United States Department of Agriculture (USDA) updated the Food Guide Pyramid to reflect the newest nutritional information. The newer form of the previous pyramid is a good reference for anyone concerned with maintaining a healthy diet. The pyramid

Box **5-1**   **Talking about Food**

Determining your patient's dietary status requires careful questioning about eating habits and other issues that affect proper nutrition. The following questions should help.
- How is your appetite?
- Are you eating more or less than your normal diet?
- Does food smell as good or taste as good as it used to?
- Do you have trouble swallowing?
- Does it sometimes feel that food just will not go down?
- Do you have frequent heartburn or indigestion?
- Do you eat out frequently? What do you usually order?
- Is it hard for you to purchase or prepare foods?
- Are there foods you cannot or will not eat?
- Have you ever followed a popular weight reduction diet recommended by a friend or advertisement?
- Are you taking diet supplements? Which ones and for what reasons?

concept encourages building a diet with a base of whole grains and working to progressively smaller portions of vegetables, fruits, dairy products, and meats and meat products and includes a very small amount of the "other" group. These guidelines include an ideal balance of nutrients to provide for cell growth and repair and to supply enough energy to make it through the day. No major source of nutrients is neglected or eliminated, as all Recommended Dietary Allowances (RDAs) are covered by the guidelines. People who follow the recommendations maintain the nutrients necessary for good health. If portion size guides are followed, an ideal weight is more likely possible than if any vital group is neglected or avoided. Following some of the current fad diets that alter the pyramid balance may lead to weight loss, but studies are not complete regarding their affect on long-term health. Although studies are ongoing, and theories are constantly challenged, it appears that diets that encourage avoiding any of these nutrients ultimately fail to maintain either health or ideal weight.

More recently, in recognition of cultural diversity, food pyramids were designed for ethnic groups such as African American, Asian, and Native American. Pyramids also offer healthy food choices for older adults, children, and vegetarians. The World Health Organization (WHO) developed pyramids for other countries that offer the best nutrition based on foods locally preferred and regionally available. Within each group, and within each culture's traditions, a healthy diet is possible by following the appropriate guidelines (Table 5-1).

Also in the early 1990s, the National Dairy Council (NDC) developed nutritional guidelines to work along with the Food Guide Pyramid. This guide urges everyone to plan a diet around all five food groups and to eat a variety of foods from each group every day for the best balance. The NDC guide illustrates the types of foods acceptable in each group on the pyramid and lists the number or size of servings of each group. It illustrates the "other" category of foods that most of us enjoy but should eat only in moderation.

Table 5-1   CULTURAL AND RELIGIOUS DIETARY PRACTICES

Group	Prohibitions	Preferences/Requirements
Catholics	Fast or abstain on certain holy days	
Hindus	Range widely from prohibiting all meats and animal products to more lenient practices	Yogurt, beans/peas, prefer to balance hot with cold and sweet with sour
Islamic/Muslims	Pork, alcohol and its products (includes alcohol-based medications), shortening made from animal products, gelatin made from animal products	
Jews	Pork, shellfish, and scavenger seafood (shrimp, crab, catfish), milk and meat dishes together, blood or bloody products, such as rare meat or blood sausage	Fish with fins and scales, Kosher products
Mainline Protestants	May forbid alcohol or tobacco, may fast for certain occasions	
Mormons	Alcohol, tobacco, and stimulant beverages (colas, coffee, tea)	
Seventh Day Adventists	Pork, shellfish, and certain other seafood, fermented beverages	

At about the same time the guidelines and pyramids were undergoing revisions and updates, the government initiated an important guide for outlining nutritional information on food labels to inform the public regarding healthy food choices. Labels on food containers must list the ingredients in the order of most abundant to least abundant, as well as additives or preservatives. Calories, fat grams, sodium, and so forth, are listed based on an average serving size (e.g., one cup, four slices). If vitamins or minerals are included, the amount compared to the RDA is also displayed. If you eat more or less than the listed serving size, the nutrient amounts must be adjusted accordingly. For example, if the label gives values for one cookie and you eat two, you must double the listed calories and other ingredients. One of the most important steps in following a prudent diet is learning to read the information posted on labels and calculating which serving options will promote health.

The recommended guidelines for a healthy diet are not hard to understand or to follow, but people with long-term poor eating habits will need your help getting started. General guidelines and suggestions follow "Healthy Nutrition for Everyone" later in this chapter. To help patients understand how to adapt the recommendations of the USDA and NDC, begin with the following suggestions:

• Teach patients to eat sensibly using foods from all food groups. Diets that eliminate any food group in the food guide pyramid may not promote long-term health. Following the recommended guidelines should lead to weight loss without compromising health.

- Whole grains, raw vegetables, and dark, rough grain breads are good diet choices. These foods are filled with vitamins, minerals, and roughage, rather than empty calories.
- Low-fat products are better choices than full-fat products, but help patients learn to read labels. Sugar may have replaced a portion of the fat, making the calorie count even higher than it would have been with the small amount of replaced fat.
- Caution patients to limit prepackaged sauce and seasoning mixes, canned soups, packaged deli meats, and frozen meals. The fat and calorie content of these items is usually very high. Teach patients to read labels; the entire RDA of fat and sodium may be found in just one serving of some foods.
- When estimating serving sizes not listed on labels as one slice, two chips, and so on, show patients how to use the following guide: 1 ounce is thumb-sized, 3 ounces are about palm-sized, a cupped hand holds about 2 liquid ounces, and a fist is about 1 cup.

Just What the Doctor Ordered

Patients who need strictly regulated diets usually are referred to nutritionists or dietitians for a full explanation that covers issues such as the reasons for the diet, the restrictions, the preferred manner of preparation, and so forth. Patients requiring long-term weight reduction, cholesterol management, or diabetic training should be under the direction of a diet specialist. Other special diets include low-calorie, low-carbohydrate, high-carbohydrate, low-fat, and low-sodium. Each of these requires more intensive training and understanding than is available to most health care professionals. Since altering intake of any of the critical nutrients is dangerous if the patient does not understand how to adjust for the change, this usually is not in the scope of training for health professions other than those specializing in diet therapy. Patient education material may cover these somewhat, but long-term diets require professional guidance. However, at times you may need to clarify instructions for an altered or modified diet ordered by the physician for short-term treatment. Those listed below usually address a critical issue such as postoperative recovery or acute gastrointestinal (GI) upset, and are not for long-term management.

In order of restriction, modified diets ordered by physicians include the following:

- *Nothing by mouth* (NPO) is not a diet; it is a method of ensuring that the GI tract is empty for procedures such as surgery or GI diagnostic studies. It is also used to rest the tract after a serious illness with vomiting and diarrhea. Unless nutrients are supplied by intravenous methods, patients should not remain NPO for long periods of time.
- *Clear liquid* diets include foods without residue that are liquid at room or body temperature, such as broth, clear juices (no pulp), gelatin, plain coffee or tea, and certain carbonated beverages. This is usually the first diet ordered as patients progress through the postoperative period or after a severe GI upset. Since this diet contains very few nutrients, patients should progress to the next level as soon as possible.
- *Full liquid* diets contain foods based on milk products, soft grains, egg products, fruit juices, and any item included in the clear liquid diet. This is a natural progression from a clear liquid diet when patients are well enough to tolerate heavier food. This diet contains more nutrients than the more restrictive levels but should not be used for long-term management.
- *Pureed diets* may be a regular diet that is processed in a blender or food processor to eliminate fiber to make it easy to swallow without chewing. It is important to make this type of diet as appealing as possible since much of our appetite and pleasure from food comes

from eye appeal and texture. This diet can be equally nutritious as a regular diet if the patient must stay on it for long-term management.

- *Soft diets* contain foods from a full liquid diet and from a regular diet. Foods must be easy to chew and digest and must be low in fiber, fat, and seasonings. Soft diets are ordered for patients who can progress from a full liquid or pureed diet but are not ready to chew or swallow a regular diet.
- *BRAT* (bananas, rice, applesauce, and toast) is prescribed for pediatric patients with diarrhea and vomiting. It is nutritious, but the child should progress to a full, age-appropriate diet as soon as possible.

All of these diets must be structured around cultural and religious restrictions and personal likes and dislikes. No amount of dietary education will work if the patient either cannot or will not eat as ordered. Determining whether the patient and caregivers understand the importance of staying within guidelines for special diets may be your responsibility. Have brochures and pamphlets on hand to describe and illustrate what is and is not allowed on the diet until the patient is ready again for a complete diet. If the patient is to remain on a restricted diet for a long time, a referral should be made to a diet specialist.

Educating Diabetic Patients

Review your appropriate texts for in-depth understanding of the physiology and pathophysiology of both type 1 diabetes mellitus (formerly referred to insulin-dependent diabetes mellitus) and type 2 diabetes mellitus (formerly known as non–insulin-dependent diabetes mellitus). Type 1 diabetes mellitus requires supplementary insulin injections to compensate for low insulin levels, usually from poorly functioning Islets of Langerhans' cells in the pancreas. Type 2 diabetes mellitus in the early stages can be controlled with diet and exercise and results when cells cannot respond to signals from available insulin to take in circulating glucose. If insulin is present in the body, but the cells are resistant, oral medication is available to help instruct cells to absorb excess glucose to lower blood sugar. Both types are chronic disorders and neither can be cured at this time, but both are manageable with proper training and understanding of the interdependence between diet, energy expenditure, and medication.

The American Diabetic Association established a model of food **exchanges** for diabetic patients to follow to help in the delicate balance between food intake and energy output. Food is divided into groups similar to the Food Guide Pyramid levels. These exchange groups allow patients to choose foods from each group in the quantity recommended by the physician to balance glucose intake and available or prescribed insulin. The balance is so delicate that patients may need to weigh each gram of food until they can accurately estimate amounts by sight. In the early stages of adjustment, dietitians spend as much time as needed to explain to patients how to manage food intake, as physicians work to determine the proper quantities of insulin for patients or caregivers to administer on an exact schedule. Patients must understand that they have to eat exactly the groups and amounts ordered by the physician and may never add or delete any food group listed for the meal. Skipping meals or adding or omitting portions can lead to serious imbalances between insulin and glucose levels.

Depending on your specialty, you may help patients understand the methods and importance of insulin administration, how to check for sores that will not heal, and how to recognize an approaching imbalance, but you probably will not be responsible for diet training. Training for the life-time management of either form, especially type 1 diabetes mellitus, requires intensive education by dietary specialists. However, as with all patient education and communication, the entire health care team must reinforce compliance and answer any questions to avoid the extensive, life-threatening complications associated with diabetes.

Eating Disorders

Much of our socialization revolves around food ("Let's meet for lunch," "Join us for dinner," or "Come over and we'll cook out"). Special food turns an everyday event into a celebration. Food plays a large part in stress management, either by increasing or decreasing intake when we are stressed, and is an escape from boredom, loneliness, and depression. Children quickly learn to use food in a power play with their parents.

All of this concentration on food leads to several food-related disorders that we see in medical practice.

- *Anorexia nervosa:* Patients with this disorder have such a distorted body image that they see themselves as obese no matter how thin they are. Bulimia (described below) may or may not be present. The disorder usually begins in the mid-teens and is found almost exclusively in cultures with plenty of available food but which value thinness as a sign of beauty and high achievement. The majority of the patients are women. Signs of anorexia nervosa include a weight loss of 25% or more for no apparent reason, with a perceived need to lose even more weight. Starvation may progress to death in up to 15% of the patients. Treatment may require psychiatric hospitalization if the patient's condition cannot be controlled in the outpatient setting. (Note: The term *anorexia* means "lack of appetite." Anorexia is usually the result of illness. *Anorexia nervosa* refers to a psychological abnormality in body image perception.)

- *Bulimia nervosa* (also known as binge and purge): Patients usually are aware that this is not normal behavior but are powerless to change it. Bulimics are usually women and girls from families that expect a high degree of success. Unlike the anorexia nervosa patient, bulimics may maintain a normal weight even though they consume large amounts of food. After eating, they usually induce vomiting and/or purge with laxatives. Obsession with weight and body image are clues, as are foul breath and tooth decay from regurgitated stomach acids. Treatment focuses on breaking the cycle and helping patients come to terms with the stress caused by the need for perfection.

- *Compulsive overeating:* Patients with the direct opposite of the above eating disorders are those whose eating habits result in obesity with weight 20% or more above the ideal for their frame. Obesity increases the risk of both forms of diabetes mellitus, hypertension, and complications from surgery or pregnancy. Depression is high among overweight patients because of our society's emphasis on thinness. Some patients have organic reasons for their overweight, such as genetic predisposition and certain endocrine disorders. However, many others use food as an escape from stress or simply do not understand the need to balance the intake of calories with an output of energy. Treatment requires lifelong behavior modification, usually under the care of a professional therapist if the overeating has a psychological basis. Patients with no contributing health problems who blame any factor other than their own behavior rarely change their destructive eating habits. Unfortunately, fewer than 30% of patients with personality-related obesity achieve and maintain an appropriate weight for very long.

Gaining control of any of the eating disorders is a life-long struggle, but so is any other long-term illness such as diabetes or heart disease, and all can be handled with proper management and education leading to changes in lifestyle behaviors.

Adjusting for a Vegetarian Lifestyle

You may at some point in your career work with patients who have chosen to eliminate animal-based protein from their diet. To help them achieve a healthy and balanced diet, you must understand the degrees of restriction in vegetarian diets and some of the basic concepts necessary to communicate knowledgeably during patient education. These diets include the following, from least restrictive to most restrictive:

- Semi-vegetarians may eat poultry, fish, and dairy products but usually will not eat pork, beef, or other red meat.
- Macrobiotic vegetarians eat whole grains, vegetables, and seafood (usually fish products) but will not eat processed food.
- Lacto-ovo vegetarians eat vegetables, dairy products, and eggs.
- Lacto-vegetarians may use milk-based products but will not eat eggs.
- Vegans eat only plant-based foods.

Patients must understand that it is important to balance protein food sources in the absence of animal protein. Most animal protein fits the body's needs completely and is readily available for metabolism; most vegetable sources are incomplete proteins and must be converted by the body to be used for growth and repair. Knowing the right combinations of incomplete proteins to supply the body's complete needs requires carefully juggling recipes. For example, cereals, nuts, most starchy vegetables, and legumes such as peas and beans are incomplete proteins. When these are combined with other complementary protein sources, such as corn or dried beans, the combination creates a complete protein. Our foremothers determined, possibly by trial and error, that recipes such as butterbeans and corn, beans and rice, corn tortillas and refried beans, bread and cheese, and so forth, were healthy for their families when meat was scarce. Even cereal and milk, a breakfast tradition, combine for a full protein source. Virtually every ethnic culture has recipes incorporating this concept. Since steady sources of meat have been available for the majority only in the past hundred or so years, all cultures adjusted by supplementing meat-based biological needs with combinations of incomplete proteins. Now that we know how the body uses proteins, we know why these combinations worked so well.

If your patient decides to limit or eliminate meat, suggest these guidelines:

- Rather than expecting the body to adjust to an immediate withdrawal of its usual protein source, the patient should phase meat out gradually. Initially, meat should be limited to one meal with meat per day, then one meat meal every 2 days, and so forth, until the body adjusts.
- Meat can be replaced or eliminated in many recipes; for example, vegetarian chili, marinara spaghetti sauce, stewed vegetables without meat.
- Grains, peas and beans, and other sources of fiber should be increased gradually. All are good sources of essential vitamins and minerals. However, if the quantity is increased too quickly, the increase in fiber may cause gastrointestinal distress.
- In the absence of meat, the diet should include a variety of foods. French fries and macaroni and cheese are vegetarian, but a steady diet of heavy fats is less healthy than one that includes red meat.
- Vegetarians should choose fortified products. Many vegetarian diets are low in certain vital nutrients, such as vitamin B12.
- Consider age and sex when structuring a diet. Women and children must supplement calcium intake to ensure bone health. Women of child-bearing age must increase iron intake.

A vegetarian diet can meet all dietary needs if all nutritional factors are carefully considered. For example, nuts and tofu safely replace the two to three servings of meat in the food guide pyramid. If milk is not included, calcium can be supplied by soy products. Many information sources are available to help those serious about eliminating animal-based foods from their diet.

Healthy Nutrition for Everyone

Good nutrition is available to most of our patients, and even those in lower socioeconomic levels will save money if they learn to shop and cook properly. Most healthy adults know how they should eat to stay healthy and probably will not be severely affected if they slip into bad habits occasionally. However, older adults and children need special considerations to protect their health.

Older adults usually have at least one of the following problems that interfere with good nutrition:

- Slowing gastrointestinal function that delays elimination and increases indigestion
- Poor dental care or poorly fitting dentures that make chewing difficult or painful
- Decrease in the sense of smell and taste leading to poor appetite
- An increased incidence of gastroesophageal reflux disease that brings food and acids from the stomach back to the esophagus, leading to pain and erosion (eating away) of the lining of the esophagus
- Depression and loneliness, making mealtime less enjoyable
- Low income, making good food choices difficult
- Multidrug interaction with foods, increasing indigestion and decreasing appetite

Older adults who do not eat well are more likely frail and fragile and also may be confused and depressed. The multiple stressors of illnesses and many medications decrease appetite, may cause nausea, and reduce the absorption of nutrients. Older adults need variety in easily digested food with pleasing texture, taste, and appearance. As eager to eat as you may be at times, think how you would feel if you were offered a plate of pureed food with no seasonings, no texture, and no visual appeal. Offer older adults and their caregivers brochures with nutrition tips for diets directed at the unique needs of the older population. Look into services such as Meals on Wheels and senior citizens centers to ensure that patients have at least one good meal per day. Helping your older patients learn to record a food diary may alert the physician to potential problems with food intake.

Children should learn early to make healthy food choices. Advise parents to offer nutritious choices in small servings and consider the size of a child's stomach. A child's stomach is just a bit larger than his fist, and that is all the food he needs at one time. Small, frequent meals are better for children than the three large meals that adults usually eat. Children burn food faster, so they need to eat more frequently. Nutritious snacks such as yogurt, cheese, and small bits of fruit or vegetables (be cautious of choking) will fill in the mealtime gaps. Advise parents to introduce children to interesting new foods pleasingly presented and they will be intrigued enough to try the foods, unless they are pressured to eat and recognize that this may be an important issue. Children and parents frequently use food as a power struggle. Many good child-rearing books outline methods to defuse the food situation in the early years before it becomes a long-term problem. Food should never be used as a reward and should never be withheld as a punishment.

Encourage low-income families with children to apply for Women, Infants and Children (WIC) funds for good nutrition. Food stamps and school lunch programs also ensure that children have a better chance for good food choices.

The following tips can be used by anyone serious about improving nutrition and adopting a healthy lifestyle.

- Encourage patients to maintain good dental health. Food is easier to eat and feels better in the mouth with real teeth rather than dentures. Overall health will improve with better dental health and hygiene.
- Teach patients how to keep a food diary for at least a week; a month is even better. Tell them to be honest about the serving sizes. Help them calculate their calories and fat grams against the recommended intake.
- Encourage patients to slow down and concentrate on the meal, rather than reading or watching TV while eating. Meals should not be eaten on the run or while doing other things.
- Teach patients to fill a small plate with small to moderate amounts of good-quality, healthy food; empty space on a large plate looks as if it should be filled. Urge dieters not to go back for seconds.
- Caution dieters not to eat out of boredom, depression, or anger. Encourage them to take a walk or ride a bike instead.
- Tell patients they should expect to lose weight slowly. Losing weight too quickly is not safe for good health and usually leads to regaining it just as quickly.
- Dieters should resist buying junk food; if it is not close at hand, impulse snacking is less likely.
- Caution dieters that caffeine intake should be kept to less than 200 to 300 mg per day. One cup of coffee has about 100 mg of caffeine and most soft drinks have comparable amounts.
- Encourage dieters to bake, broil, grill, or saute lean meats, poultry, and fish rather than frying.
- Using herbs and spices rather than salt, fat, or sauces highlights the taste of food without adding calories or fat.
- Six to eight glasses of water a day keeps tissues hydrated and helps elimination. A large glass of water before a meal may help the dieter eat less.
- Skipping meals is not a good idea. The dieter usually will eat more at the next meal or fill up on junk food.

Teach patients to focus on a healthy diet, balanced by exercise, rather than concentrating entirely on weight reduction. Wellness should be the goal, not someone's idea of an ideal weight. These guidelines will not make the dieter model-thin but will lead to better health.

EXERCISING FOR HEALTH

A balanced, nutritious diet improves or maintains health for all age groups. However, the greatest benefits are gained from a combination of proper diet—the intake of nutrients—and the best possible fitness routine—the output of calories. It is possible to lose weight and stay healthy from diet alone, but adding **exercise** to a healthy diet increases the benefits many times over. Exercise makes us look better and feel better as it makes our heart and lungs more efficient and improves blood pressure, heart rate, and cardiac patterns. It lowers cholesterol and blood sugar levels and increases immune cell function. Sustained movement relieves stress and tension and improves our mood and thought processes. It helps us lose weight or maintain an ideal weight, decreases hunger, and increases metabolism and elimination. Exercise strengthens muscles and bones and improves flexibility, posture, and energy. Every system works at peak efficiency when we are physically fit.

Exercise is natural. Watch babies stretch and kick and move every muscle, or try to keep up with a toddler's constant motion. From birth through old age, our bodies need to move and will deteriorate when forced to remain still. We see this in patients confined to bed rest who develop clots, weakened bones, and wasted muscles. Those who choose to be sedentary grow obese; develop hypertension, diabetes, and heart disease; and are more likely to be depressed. Children who are not allowed to play outside, perhaps for safety reasons, are less likely to develop strong bones or reach a full growth potential and are more likely to be obese throughout life. Technology has taken over much of our need to move about. What was once done by manual or physical labor is now done by machine, but the need to exercise is still a strong physiological goal, unless we subdue it until exercise no longer seems natural. We learn very early to be either active or sedentary.

There are many obstacles to exercise. Patients who are already ill may not be able to exercise because of factors such as degenerative joint disease, multiple sclerosis, Parkinson's disease, or the side effects of medications. The chronic stresses of illness or difficult life situations are exhausting and depressing, which makes it harder to gather the energy needed for exercise. Many of our patients live in areas unsafe for outside activity but cannot afford to join health clubs. If patients are physically able to exercise, encourage them to look through the day for constructive ways to expend energy rather than taking the lazy way. Exercise can be included in many everyday activities. Encourage patients to walk around the block rather than eating junk food, climb the stairs rather than waiting for the elevator, park far from the shop door rather than looking for the closest parking space, and walk briskly rather than ambling along. Although several weekly sessions of sustained activity work best, exercise does not have to take place in organized aerobic classes.

Several types and combinations of beneficial movements make up recognized exercise regimens. These include the following:

- *Isokinetic exercise* uses muscle contraction against resistance, such as lifting weights through a **range of motion** (ROM). Many of the structured programs using exercise machines are designed to work each muscle group to the best advantage for strengthening or endurance.
- *Isometric exercise* causes muscle contraction without shortening the joint angle. This includes pushing on an object with the arms stiffened. The muscle contracts, but the joint angle stays the same. This form of exercise strengthens muscles and increases blood flow to a part.
- *Isotonic exercise* shortens or contracts muscles and creates movement at the joint. A good example is a biceps curl, especially with weights. Isotonic movements include walking, jogging, and cycling. These movements improve cardiopulmonary function and increase strength and muscle mass.

Programs such as aerobics, strength or endurance training, and stretching or flexibility programs include many of these exercise concepts. Aerobic exercises require sustained motions, usually rhythmic, that increase metabolism to burn calories, improve heart and lung function, and increase the muscle to fat ratio. Swimming, jogging, walking, and dancing are good examples. Strength or endurance training includes weight training with free weights or stack systems, calisthenics, and isometric movements. Stretching through the range of motion improves flexibility and posture and is included in many forms of yoga and dance. Trainers and instructors help clients learn to move muscles to the best advantage to avoid injury. If a professional trainer is not within a patient's budget, good training books

Box **5-2**   **Talking about Exercise**

To determine if the patient is ready for an exercise program, and to assist the physician in deciding which program is best, ask questions such as the following:

- Do you fit exercise into your day, either in your job or for fun? How much? What type?
- Is your job generally active or usually sedentary?
- Does physical activity cause dizziness or shortness of breath? Does it cause chest pain?
- Are you on any medications that may cause you to be dizzy or weak?
- Do you fall frequently or are you afraid you might fall?
- Does any specific movement cause joint or muscle pain? Can you describe the movement and the pain?
- Do you have health problems that keep you from exercising, such as angina, asthma, or joint pain?
- Do you feel safe exercising outside? For instance, do you live in a safe neighborhood or have an area for exercising where there is a low risk for falls?
- Has your mobility recently gotten better or worse? Can you describe any changes in mobility?

are available at most bookstores to explain the movements and encourage safety. Any well-rounded exercise plan includes some sort of aerobic activity, strengthening exercises, and flexibility routine.

Patients who have been inactive or have not exercised for a while should consult their physician before beginning an exercise program (Box 5-2). If the patient is older than 35 years and has been generally sedentary, an exercise physiologist recommended by the physician will plan a course for the greatest advantage with the lowest risk of injury. Physicians are usually delighted when patients begin to practice prudent lifestyle behaviors but may have reservations and recommendations for patients with fragile health. A medically oriented program and professionally trained instructor help protect sedentary or unhealthy persons from injury and make it more likely that the patient will continue the program.

For patient education material, have brochures on hand from reputable programs such as the American Heart Association. All good exercise resources offer routines for individual ability and explain the proper movement to avoid injury. The following suggestions will help ensure patients exercise safely and effectively:

- Caution patients not to work through pain. Pain is a sign that something is wrong. The exerciser should slow down and make sure the motion is being performed properly.
- Advise the exerciser to slow down if he or she has trouble talking or breathing. Oxygen intake and proper breathing techniques are very important in exercise routines.
- Help patients determine a target heart rate using an acceptable, age-adjusted scale. Patients usually should stay within their safest range.
- Advise patients to drink plenty of water before, during, and after exercise.
- Exercisers should warm up for 5 to 10 minutes before increasing the energy level and slow down, or cool down, after the exercise for the same amount of time. The pace should be gradually increased to a proper sustained level, then slowed to end the exercise. It is not safe to stop a workout abruptly.
- Muscles should be stretched slowly during warm-up and cool-down to release muscle fibers. Stretches should be held for at least a count of 10.

- Everyone should stretch all during the day as they move about. Cats and dogs have the right idea; they stretch whenever they change positions.
- It is not necessary to use expensive weights or equipment. Inexpensive flexible bands work as resistance for good, safe routines.
- Suggest that exercisers choose a partner. When one is not in the mood, the other can be the motivator.
- If a health club is too expensive, a good pair of shoes and a brisk walk is a good substitute.
- Suggest activities the exerciser will enjoy. If exercise is fun, we are more likely to stick with it.
- Help the exerciser set goals—one more block, 5 more minutes, three more repetitions.
- Help patients keep a record and praise them when they reach their goal.

Patients who cannot exercise because of illness or injury need help to maintain muscle function. Even those who are not expected to regain full function should work through a full range of all joint movements for prescribed periods to prevent musculoskeletal problems. These include loss of bone density, shortening of muscle fibers (called contractures), and a decrease in blood and nerve supply to tissues leading to pressure ulcers. Passive range of motion exercises (PROM) performed by a professional or a caregiver help prevent these complications. Since this is time-consuming and requires skill, machines can be used to move a limb through a PROM until the patient is able to perform the exercise without assistance. If these skills are within your scope of practice, they will be covered in your clinical texts.

THE STRESS FACTOR

It is not so much stress itself that leads to physical or mental illness: the problem lies with how we handle stress. Our physical and mental resources, coping mechanisms (covered later in this chapter), social support, and the type and degree of stress all work together to determine how we are affected.

Although stress is usually undeniably a negative experience, certain stressful situations are positive. This is called **eustress** (**positive stress**, or good stress), such as pushing yourself to the limit for something you enjoy. Positive stress helps most people work efficiently and perform better than they might without a certain degree of pressure. In fact, many people work best under positive stress; for example, rushing around to prepare for an enjoyable anticipated event, such as a party, vacation, or holidays. However, even when these stressful situations are fun, we need time to rest when the event is over. With no time to relax, even positive stress becomes negative as we become more tired and have no time to refuel.

For this text, we generally concentrate on **negative stress**. Stress overload may be as catastrophic as war or famine or may be simply an accumulation of daily irritations (lost keys, minor arguments). We all respond to stress differently; certain types of stress for one person may not be a problem for another. For example, an action or event that stresses you (jumping out of an airplane) may be an enjoyable challenge to someone else. Responses also vary from day to day; stressors that overwhelm us today may be manageable tomorrow. A fender-bender can be aggravating and expensive, for example, but should not be devastating, unless we are already sick or stressed and feel that we cannot manage even one more burden. Great negative events or small unavoidable everyday irritations add up to too many things to handle and may lead to stress overload.

Review your anatomy and physiology or biology text to remember how the autonomic nervous system works to balance the response of its parasympathetic and sympathetic systems.

The parasympathetic system works to calm and soothe the body in an unthreatened state when there is no crisis or when a recent crisis is over. As a matter of survival, the sympathetic branch of the nervous system controls the stress response when we sense a threat. Unfortunately, the system cannot tell the difference between positive and negative stress. It handles joyful stress (such as marriage or a coveted new job) just as it does life-threatening situations. The body feels that chronic stress (a bad marriage, long-term illness), acute stress (a final exam, an interview, or a life-threatening situation), and sequential stress (a series of stressors) need the same protective mechanisms. The heart beats faster to rush oxygen and glucose to muscles to make them work more efficiently. The respiratory rate increases to supply oxygen, and glucose levels rise to supply fuel. Blood pressure rises to force blood into the tissues needed to fight or to run away. Blood rushes to the heart, lungs, and brain and flows away from the surface of the body, leaving hands and feet cold. Blood thickens to slow bleeding in case the source of stress leads to bloodshed. Pupils dilate to bring in every available visual image for processing. Digestion slows so that available energy is used for survival. All of our internal forces concentrate on dealing with whatever threatens our life or our homeostatic balance. If stress is not resolved quickly, resources are exhausted, leaving no energy to cope with additional stressors. Mild stress makes us work more efficiently and think more clearly and challenges us to grow; severe or unrelieved stress makes us sick.

Unless stress is relieved, it can lead to physical signs and symptoms such as the following:

- Headache, stiff neck, or tension in the back and shoulders
- Upset stomach, diarrhea or constipation, dry mouth and throat, difficulty swallowing
- Rapid heart rate and shortness of breath
- Anxiety that may lead to panic
- Exhaustion or lack of energy
- Disordered thoughts and poor concentration
- Loss of short-term memory
- Insomnia and nightmares

Ultimately, long-term stress leads to many illnesses. Although a genetic predisposition usually must be present to trigger most of the stress-related diseases and disorders, the presence of stress apparently overwhelms resistance and makes patients more susceptible to illnesses associated with the sympathetic response. Clearly, to keep our patients well, we must help them manage unavoidable everyday stress and the added stress of illness.

The General Adaptation Syndrome

Hans Selye, an endocrinologist, studied how the organs of secretion (the endocrine glands) respond to stress. Selye studied and documented the difference between local adaptation syndrome (LAS) and general adaptation syndrome (GAS). He described LAS as pain or inflammation after an injury and noted that the body's response is usually confined to the area of injury. Selye realized, however, that in a threatening or stressful situation, the body responds with a systemwide alert. He outlined the response as three stages:

- The alarm or appraisal stage mobilizes the body to respond to the crisis. The body tries to determine, "How threatening is this situation?" and "How much response do I need?" In this stage, the sympathetic nervous system is on full alert. Patients in this stage may be too frightened to react logically. Do not burden patients in this stage with too much unnecessary information; small, manageable bits of information are easier to process. Give patients small choices, such as which procedure to perform first, or which day or time is best for the next visit. The opportunity to make small choices helps patients regain a feeling of control. However, do not be surprised if patients have trouble making even minor decisions during this stage.

- The resistance or adaptation stage either fights against or adjusts to the stressor. The body works to restore balance or homeostasis. The sympathetic system feels it must be ready for fright/flight or fight, so all other functions are put on "hold" or "stand by" until the crisis is over. Patients wonder, "How can I handle this?" "How will this affect my physical, mental and emotional resources?" Patients are frequently angry and frustrated at this stage. Though the anger may be directed at you, do not take it personally; see this as a part of the illness and handle it with compassion and understanding as you would any other sign or symptom.

- The previous stages lead to the exhaustion stage when physical resources are depleted and there is no energy left to fight. Prolonged stress may result in psychosomatic disorders (generated in the mind) or **organic** illness with actual physical findings. All of the sympathetic responses described above take an enormous toll on the body and mind (Fig. 5-3). Be especially sensitive to signs of depression in this stage (described later in this chapter).

If we are mentally strong and otherwise healthy, we may move through stress and be stronger for having faced it. In addition to available physical resources, many social factors affect the ability to withstand a stressful situation. These include the following: Are we cared for and loved? Are our other hierarchical needs met? Can we network for information resources to help us? Do we have the financial resources to weather the crisis? All of these personal considerations ultimately affect our ability to withstand stressors both large and small.

The Stress of Illness

Stress is understandable and unavoidable in catastrophes such as war or natural disasters (tornadoes, earthquakes), or in smaller stressors, such as our many day-to-day aggravations, but for our purposes in this section, we will concentrate on the stress brought on by illness.

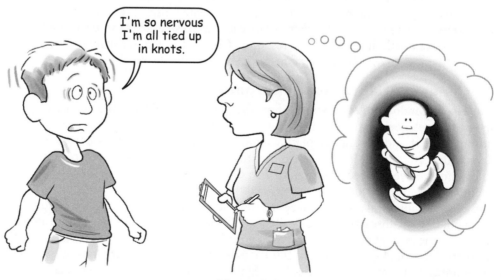

Figure 5-3

Until our more recent medical advances, many patients died before reaching the levels of illness that we now see every day. This requires not just more professional competency in health care, it also requires more understanding of the mental trauma of illness and the adjustments that patients must make in order to survive emotionally as well as physically. How patients feel about themselves changes, as they think, "I am a cardiac patient now. If I am not 'me' anymore, how can I and those who love me adjust to this new 'me'?" In general, patients must be prepared to face both physical and psychological pain as they heal, or must adjust to the fact that they may never fully recover. Some must realize that they cannot care for themselves and can no longer live independently. They may be required to endure treatments and procedures that frequently are painful and debilitating and may be long term. Their self-image, life role, and personal relationships may change to accommodate the affects of illness. All of these stressors are factors to consider during our interaction with all patients, but communication is more difficult with those who are severely ill.

All patients, no matter how slightly or severely ill, must learn a new language for the medical community with its strange and frightening customs and behaviors. Patients need answers to questions they may be afraid to ask, such as, "Can I expect pain?" "When will it become bearable, or will it always be unbearable?" "Will it ever end?" "Will I lose control of my bladder, my bowels, my mobility, and can I ever regain control?" Many questions tumble over in their minds and add to the confusion and depression associated with any illness. Most patients do better with less stress when they know what lies ahead in 2 weeks, 2 months, or 2 years. It helps to know in advance the next step in the progression of illness. Knowing what lies ahead can lead to the following:

- Seeking knowledge. When patients know the direction of the illness, some begin to research to know more about the disorder and how to handle it. With the help of family, social groups, and health care providers, many patients take control and work toward a reasonable level of wellness.
- Seeking comfort. Patients look for comfort and support from their social and spiritual groups and within the medical community. This love/belonging hierarchical need is never more important than during illness.
- Learning self-care. If the illness is extreme, patients need a strong ego and mental resources to adjust to the changes. Some changes can be devastating to the self-image, but knowing what to expect helps to prepare for self-care. Your role in this area of adjustment involves helping with procedures necessary for management of the illness.
- Goal setting. Breaking the illness into small, manageable components makes the changes more acceptable. For example, "First, we will go over what to expect with the incision, then you can learn to change the dressing."
- Planning alternative directions. Life plans may be altered to fit the new self-image and physical limitations. Patients who realize this and make realistic adjustments fairly early in the illness usually respond better throughout the illness.

Patients with acute, short-term illnesses who are expected to recover fully and rather quickly, naturally adjust more quickly and usually follow directions to speed recovery. Knowing that the illness will be long and possibly painful or debilitating leads to poor adjustment and, unfortunately, poor compliance. It is also somewhat easier to adapt with less stress to an illness that is not obvious to observers, even if it is long-term. Think of several illnesses or injuries that are difficult to hide, such as facial disfigurement, oxygen support, wheelchair or walker assistance, certain physical and mental impairments; any of these cause questioning glances or curious stares. Many other illnesses have no outward signs, such as most cardiac or endocrine disorders or skin disorders confined to the trunk; even colostomies and mastectomies are not obvious to the casual observer. These seem to be less depressing and easier on patients in social situations, since they are not usually as devastating to self-esteem as those disorders that everyone can see. Your role is to support the patient and listen when tears are near, or when there is a need to talk about the changes, challenges, and adjustments. Listen with a caring, compassionate heart, and refer patients and caregivers to support groups. It helps to talk about these things with someone who has handled the situation personally.

Relaxing for Stress Relief

Relaxing calms the stress response, relieves short-term stress, and keeps small, everyday aggravations from accumulating into large, illness-producing stressors. Several easy-to-perform relaxation techniques listed below help to regulate vital signs and put patients in a frame of mind to listen and learn. As you learn these techniques, teach them to your patients.

Most of the following examples require a mind-over-body attitude that "wills" the body to relax. This has a two-fold effect. Willing the mind to calm itself also calms the body. As the body relaxes, vital signs return to normal, stress hormone levels drop, and every system involved in the stress response works toward balance. Your patients can use these easy techniques as they wait for physical examinations or treatment procedures.

Stretching

Muscles tense during stress in preparation for a flight or fight response. In a short while, tight muscles tire from the tension, adding to the exhaustion of stress. Stretching through the whole body with hands high over the head is the easiest way to relieve muscle tension. This can be done sitting, but is more effective standing. Stretch through the shoulders, rib cage, hips and legs. Tighten every muscle group, then will them to relax. Work from the top of the head to the toes; then back again. Many good stretching exercises give a whole-body workout and are easy to do. Patients can invest in either a good class or a good instruction book to learn proper technique.

Yoga stretching exercises are very good for relieving muscle tension and can fit into small time frames for tension relief.

Breathing Deeply

Learning to breathe correctly for tension relief works in two ways: there is a better exchange of oxygen and carbon dioxide, and concentrating on breathing takes the mind off of stress.

Sit or stand with good posture (slumping interferes with respiration) with hands on the abdomen. Breathe deeply through the nose as the abdomen moves outward. Hold the breath for a few seconds and try to breathe in more deeply. Exhale through pursed lips with the hands pulling the abdomen inward toward the spine. This should be done until stress flows out with each breath.

Visualizing

Think of a better place to be—a warm, sunny beach or a cool mountaintop. Concentrate on developing the pleasant image. This is a good method of stress relief when the timing is appropriate, such as while waiting to see a doctor or just before a test.

Meditating

Setting aside as little as 5 or 10 minutes for meditation is a great stress reliever. It may be harder to relax at certain times than at others; however, rushing to relax makes it worse. Several yoga poses were developed for stress relief, but simply sitting still and quiet may help quiet the stress response. Set a timer for the target period. Focus on a word or phrase, a thought or an image. If other thoughts intrude, will them away and go back to the focus point. Do not keep checking the timer. When the time has passed, take a deep breath, stretch (both described above) and go about the day in a better frame of mind.

Exercising

The best natural tranquilizer is physical exercise (described in Exercising for Health above). Working through all of the muscle groups relieves tension and releases the body's natural mood elevators. Fitting this time into your busy schedule is one of the most important variables in a healthy lifestyle.

LEARNING TO COPE

This text is not designed to address deep psychological illnesses or abnormal psychology. Mental disorders may be covered in the pathology component of your course, while this text focuses on communicating with patients to relieve the psychological effects of illness. For our purposes, we refer to issues in response to current, acute life situations, such as illness or injury or coping with the care of someone who is ill.

The *American Heritage Dictionary* defines **coping** as "to contend (to battle) or strive, especially on even terms or with success; to contend with difficulties and act to overcome them." This definition implies that coping is a positive mechanism. Stress and tension are not necessarily negative factors; at times, they may be all that holds us together. If we do not feel natural stress in a bad situation, we cannot gather the resources to respond and make it better; however, if we are too stressed, we are equally incapable of responding. We need fewer defense or coping mechanisms (described in Box 5-3) if we have strong self-esteem and reliable social support (family and friends), but we still need ways to reduce troubling or overwhelming stressors that cannot be quickly or easily resolved. Since life is rarely stress-free, it helps to understand how the mind works consciously and subconsciously to help us react to our environment while it protects us from stress overload.

Coping Mechanisms: Defenses against Stress

The level of stress experienced depends on what the stressor means to the patient. For example, escaping from a bad marriage is very stressful, but if the change is for the better, the stress can be managed more easily than if the change in situation brings more bad than good. Patients who are facing the loss of some aspect of their "self" react depending upon the value they place on that loss. A pianist may not mind a scarred face or body but may be devastated by a loss of hand movement. An actress may not mind hands stiffened by arthritis but may grieve for the loss of beauty. The change and its stressors are the same, but the response changes with the patient's perception. Potentially stressful changes are not a major problem unless we think they are. Most of us face our problems head-on and confront challenges to change the situation into manageable components. This is easier with strong support from friends and family to relieve some of the pressure.

Some patients choose to deny or ignore that they are stressed. There is nothing basically wrong with denial in health care as a protection against stress if treatment regimens are followed. If the patient does not want to believe that she had a myocardial infarction but makes the necessary adjustments, this may be acceptable. Short-term denial helps delay facing the problem until the patient is better able to adjust to the changes. However, patients must, at some point, focus attention on coping with the situation. If she denies that her heart function is affected and will not make the necessary changes, this is inappropriate, or **maladaptive**.

Defense mechanisms or coping strategies are reinforced and re-used many times when we find the ones that work for us to reduce stress and control anxiety. Some methods are more natural for certain personalities than others. For example, patients who prefer to escape reality than face challenges may use fantasizing or denial, whereas those who tackle problems aggressively may use displacement or projection. Mechanisms we see most often in health care are listed in Box 5-3.

Understanding and recognizing coping mechanisms does not give us the depth of knowledge to analyze patients or to play amateur psychologist. However, this information may make it easier to assist patients through stressful situations.

Coping mechanisms become maladaptive when we continue to use them as an escape beyond the need to adapt to stress or if they are not effective in protecting us. Examples of maladaptive coping strategies include such things as alcohol and drugs, both of which add significantly to stressful situations. A socially acceptable form of maladaptive coping is escaping into work to avoid confronting things that should be changed. The problem has not gone away; we are just too busy and tired to see it. In health care, we also see those who assume "sick behaviors" or the "sick role" to cope with stress. This is a socially acceptable escape to gain sympathy, rest, and caring and to avoid unpleasantness, as the patient asks, "How can I deal with this problem when I am so sick?" Patients who make no effort to contribute to a return to health, or who refuse to comply with health care directives, may have chosen to protect themselves from stress by assuming the sick role. If stress is not relieved by these maladaptive coping mechanisms—and they are rarely effective—the situation will deteriorate with a breakdown in social relationships and an increase in stress.

To help our patients contend successfully with stress, encourage them to try these suggestions:

- Help them look at the situation objectively to see what they can change to make it more manageable.
- List options and possible solutions in pro and con columns. Seeing the problem on paper helps put it in perspective.
- Encourage them to be realistic. Is it as bad as it seems? What can be done to make it better? Can the patient adjust or adapt if it does not improve?
- Help them adjust their priorities. What can wait versus what must be done now?
- Help them to see that if what they are doing to resolve stress is not working, they should stop doing it and try something else. They should avoid digging themselves into a deeper hole of stress and depression.
- Stress that self-actualization goals may have to wait. Since no one can do everything at once, they must concentrate on surviving.
- Be available if patients need help finding answers to their questions. While no one has all of the answers, it is important to know where to look for answers.
- Encourage patients to say "No" when they must and to limit as many commitments as possible. Does she need to serve on so many committees or take on everyone else's responsibilities?

Box **5-3** Coping or Defense Mechanisms

The following methods of coping with stress are commonly seen in medical practice:

- Compensation: Developing strengths to overcome weaknesses. Patients with impaired vision may develop stronger hearing to compensate.
- Displacement: Striking out at a substitute, usually someone or something unable to fight back rather than the source of anger. Patients or caregivers may seem angry with you when they cannot direct their anger at the situation. For example, a caregiver may rage at you when the anger cannot be directed at the patient.
- Fantasizing: Daydreaming as a means of escape. A patient may choose a fantasy such as, "When I am well again, I will sell all of my belongings and travel around the world." This is not a bad strategy unless it interferes with adjustment.
- Humor: Laughing at ourselves or at a situation. It may be hard to find humor in most medical situations, but some patients can genuinely laugh at themselves. Imagine the patient honestly laughing at herself in an unbecoming patient gown. Laughter helps relieve stress.
- Projection: Blaming someone else for one's own behavior. Every bad choice is someone else's fault, since it is easier to blame others. Abusers and alcoholics frequently blame someone else for their own unacceptable behavior.
- Rationalization: Justifying a behavior or situation by deceiving ourselves into thinking it is acceptable. An example is the smoker who thinks, "I will have to die of something, I may as well enjoy myself."
- Regression: Returning to an earlier developmental stage as an escape from stress. Patients may regress to tantrums, pouting, and other childish behaviors to get what they want or to avoid facing stressful decisions. Children frequently drop back to an earlier stage during illness or stress.
- Repression: Involuntarily rejecting painful thoughts and realities from the conscious mind. Victims of child abuse and survivors of traumatic experiences sometimes protect themselves by storing the memories so deeply that it may take years of intensive psychotherapy to bring them back to a conscious level. Repressed memories and unacknowledged anger can lead to a number of mental or physical illnesses.
- Suppression: Deliberately refusing to acknowledge something that causes mental pain or suffering. As opposed to regression, these patients consciously delay thinking painful thoughts or facing difficult decisions until they feel strong enough to face reality. This reaction, like denial, may be appropriate if it does not interfere with health care.
- Undoing: Making amends; attempting to cancel out an unacceptable behavior by one that is more acceptable. Patients may think, "I was angry at her earlier, so I will be extra nice this time."

- Help them recognize that stress is inevitable. Help them plan that stress will happen and encourage them that eventually they will cope with it successfully.
- Help them have a plan B in case plan A does not work.
- Encourage them to look for respite to rest their mind, such as music, friends, or happy entertainment, and to avoid depressing people or situations as much as possible.
- Help patients to laugh often and stay positive. Negativity increases stress.
- Show patients how to help someone else when they are able. Support groups depend on all of the members to help each other, which helps each member concentrate less on himself.

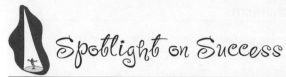

Spotlight on Success

> Dealing with the death of a patient is often one of the most stressful moments in your career, especially if you were directly involved in performing emergency care. Many hospitals and communities offer critical incident stress debriefing programs (CISD). CISD programs help health care professionals deal with the stress felt following a critical incident whether it was an in-hospital event or from an outside setting. You can find CISD professionals by calling your local hospital or through the Internet. To have a long and successful career in health care you will need to find ways to manage stressful events.

- Encourage patients to exercise within their limits, eat right, and take care of themselves.
- Encourage patients to turn to their spiritual guide (pastor, rabbi, or priest) for hope and encouragement.
- Let them be angry if they must, but help them look for acceptable outlets and move beyond it.

These tips may help your patients regain control over challenges and stressors. Remember, the problem is still there—the challenge is to meet the needs of the situation and to build protection from psychological as well as physiological stress (see Spotlight on Success box).

Managing Depression: When Coping Mechanisms Do Not Work

Depression occurs when coping mechanisms are not effective or when we are not emotionally or psychologically strong enough to contend with stress. Depression can also be a coping mechanism if we withdraw from the situation and leave decision-making to others. A seriously depressed patient probably will not follow a health regimen and more likely will increase the risk of illness.

Depression is defined as a deep unhappiness and is characterized by hopelessness, despair, a negative outlook, lethargy, and a feeling of worthlessness. It may be acute, and never happen again (this is situational and usually improves when the situation is corrected), or may recur at intervals. Variations and degrees of depression affect almost everyone at some point. Studies show that more women than men suffer from depression; it peaks in the middle years between 20 to 60 years, at about 40 years of age, and affects fewer very young and very old than the middle-age groups. More women confess that they are depressed and seek help; more men act out depression in violence or self-destructive behavior.

Symptoms should be present for at least 2 weeks for a diagnosis of depression to be made. Signs and symptoms include those listed above and the following:

- Loss of interest in normal activities and occupations. Patients who are normally pleasant and well groomed may be irritable and poorly dressed. School and job absences are common, home responsibilities and hobbies are ignored, and social obligations are neglected.
- Changes in sleeping and/or eating patterns, either more or less. Some patients avoid sleep to avoid disturbing dreams, which leads to exhaustion and further depression; others sleep excessively to avoid coping with stress. Some people eat to fill the emptiness; others have no appetite and have trouble swallowing.

- Altered activity patterns, either hyperactive or sluggish. Normally active people complain of no energy, normally placid people rush around in a panic.
- A feeling of guilt or worthlessness for no apparent reason. Some depressed patients feel guilty and worry that they are not worth the attention the depression brings.
- An inability to concentrate or to think clearly. Managing depression overwhelms thought processes; there is nothing left for normal thought patterns.

Endogenous ("beginning within") depression has either a physical or psychological basis rather than situational, or **exogenous**, depression that occurs in response to an outside source of stress. Endogenous depression may be associated with the polar disorders, bipolar and unipolar. The **manic**, or hyperactive, stage of bipolar disorder is characterized by feelings of **euphoria** and **invincibility**, as patients feel they are on top of the world and can do anything they wish; they feel they simply cannot fail. Stages then range through periods of normal behavior and emotions to possibly feeling "blue," then may deteriorate to severe, almost **catatonic** depression requiring hospitalization as the patient can scarcely move or function. Unipolar patients are frequently symptom-free with normal emotional levels until the disorder becomes dominant. This is referred to as major depression. Unipolar depression is different from bipolar in that there is no manic state. Either polar disorder requires a careful balance of psychotropic agents (mind-altering medications) and psychiatric care and usually must be treated for life. Several theories are at odds for the cause of endogenous depression and include the following:

- Biological factors relating to a chemical imbalance in the brain, possibly inherited.
- Psychological interference based on repressed memories and conflicts. The repressed memories may be struggling to surface.
- A tendency to view life experiences negatively; this is usually a learned response. In other words, these people were taught to see every occurrence in the worst possible light.

Less debilitating forms of endogenous depression include premenstrual syndrome (PMS), postpartum depression, menopausal depression, and seasonal affective disorder (SAD) (winter blues, cabin fever). If these forms do not resolve on their own, mild mood elevators, exercise, diet, and sunlight seem to help. If these forms become severe, they may require psychotherapy and psychotropic medications. Most endogenous depression has little to do with the actual degree of stress present and may appear for no apparent reason.

We are more likely to see reactive or situational depression in general medical practices other than psychiatry. This form of depression is exogenous and is the result of a life event. It is considered an adjustment disorder or inability to adjust to a current stressor. It is usually short term and is linked to something happening currently or to a remembered situation, such as the anniversary of a significant loss. These patients need a strong support network and may need a mild mood elevator to help them through the crisis. Help them talk and grieve for relief. This form of depression usually resolves in time.

Depression, like a fever, is not a disease but a symptom. It tells us that something is wrong but does not tell us what. If time, caring, and compassion are not enough to relieve the underlying cause, professional psychiatric or psychological care may determine the origin and lead to appropriate treatment.

Understanding Suicide

The ultimate failure at coping is suicide. It is hard for us to accept that someone would choose to end his life while others work so hard to live. This person needs our help to live as surely as someone with a physical illness. Suicide leaves a wide circle of bereavement with dynamics different from those of normal grief. The survivor guilt can be devastating, as family members and friends wonder why their caring was not enough and why they did not see the signs.

You should be aware of several facts about suicide to alert you to high-risk situations.

• Many patients considering suicide talk about it, but some do not. If a patient mentions that she is thinking about suicide, she probably means it.

• Suicide as a way to handle stress runs in families. If one member has killed himself, be alert for other members.

• Most suicidal patients are undecided and tempt fate to save them. Patients may think, "If someone comes and wakes me from these sleeping pills, I wasn't meant to die." Teens and young children usually fall in this category, and their numbers are rising.

• The impulse to end one's life comes and goes. The urge is rarely consistent.

• Suicide numbers rise around holidays, possibly when loneliness and forced gaiety are hardest to handle.

• Depressives are more likely to kill themselves as they withdraw from deep depression than while they are in the deepest stages. They usually lack the strength while they are most depressed and will do anything to never sink to those depths of mental anguish again.

• Bipolar manic-depressive patients may be more susceptible to suicide as they come down from a manic high.

• Older adults are more likely to think through the process and are usually more successful than younger people, who may act more impulsively.

• More women than men attempt suicide; more men than women are successful.

• Elderly white men who have suffered several losses are most likely to attempt suicide and are usually most successful.

• Certain cultures honor and expect suicide as an admirable solution to loss of respect or as a response to tragedy.

• Sometimes, if the means of suicide seems particularly painful, physical pain may be preferred to the emotional pain of depression. Some methods of suicide are an effort to finally feel something other than mental anguish.

• Watch for hoarding medication, giving away treasured items, a sudden decision to donate body parts, asking for forgiveness, settling old debts, and statements regarding "ending it all."

At any time that you suspect a patient is suicidal, discuss your concern with the physician. Be there to listen to the patient as she discusses her life and why she is so unhappy. Ask directly, "Are you thinking about suicide?" If she is not, her cues should tell you that she is surprised by the question. If she is thinking of suicide, watch for cues of avoiding the subject; more likely, however, she will be relieved that she can talk to you. It does not work to simply tell a potential suicide that this is wrong. Many fear pain, suffering, and dependence more than death. Encourage patients to talk with the physician, who probably will refer them to a professional for help through this devastatingly painful time.

An aspect of suicide that we must consider in noncompliant patients is passive suicide. These patients do not actively pursue suicide like those who swallow too many pills or shoot themselves; they simply do not do anything to help themselves live. They practice risky behavior, stop taking vital medications, ignore treatment directions, and so on. Not every patient who does this is working toward suicide, of course. Many other factors must be considered before approaching the patient with questions about his or her intentions. In many situations with these behaviors, patients did not understand the importance of the treatment options, which gives you another opportunity to stress patient education.

THE IMPACT OF SUBSTANCE ABUSE AND ADDICTION

With the abundance of illegal drugs available, you will work with patients affected by substance abuse and addiction at some point in your career. Substance abuse in any form is a grave concern, but addiction has a profound impact on family dynamics, health care, and society in general. In this section, we are concerned with understanding the physical and mental health impact of substance abuse and addiction. Understanding is always the first step in making any interaction more productive.

Addiction is defined as either physiological or psychological dependence on a substance or practice beyond voluntary control. Physiological addiction affects body chemistry at such a deep level and to such an extent that withdrawing the substance produces a reaction at the cellular level, sometimes causing severe complications. Persons most likely to develop a physiological addiction may be biologically susceptible to certain substances, such as alcohol or nicotine. They seem to metabolize the chemicals differently than others who use, but do not abuse, potentially addicting chemicals. The susceptibly addictive person may be addicted after brief exposure to a substance that others can use occasionally without developing an addiction.

If addiction does not involve a biologically based need, the substance may be used as an escape from stress or to alter an unpleasant reality and may be made more intense by the person's psychology, culture, or a combination of factors. Studies suggest that addictive personalities usually have a low frustration threshold and poor self-esteem and need the support of the substance as a coping mechanism. People who are psychologically addicted may be so attached to this form of stress relief that they subconsciously increase stress levels as an excuse to fall back into the behavior. For example, the smoker or alcoholic who is trying to stop, but starts a fight with a spouse as an excuse to say, "See, you made me start smoking (or drinking) again when I was trying so hard to stop." (Both alcohol and nicotine are usually physiologically addicting.) Addictive personalities may not be physiologically addicted and usually do not suffer the same physical symptoms on withdrawal. These persons need to develop coping skills rather than resorting to chemical substances as a defense mechanism. Psychological addiction, also called habituation, becomes a habit and is seen in people who function better in social situations with a cigarette and drink in hand to overcome awkwardness but may not need the substances at other times.

Patients affected by alcohol or other commonly abused substances should be under the supervision of trained specialists. Problems of this significance require careful assessment and management and probably are not within your scope of practice. However, because the abuse of addictive substances has such a profound effect on health, take every opportunity to provide patients with education and access to support groups.

Every substance listed in Box 5-4 is dangerous to the substance abuser; however, they also have strong adverse and potentially deadly effects during pregnancy. Fetal alcohol syndrome is well documented, and for certain metabolisms, even a small amount of maternal alcohol intake may result in fetal damage. Even second-hand smoke has been shown to affect the fetus. Pregnant substance abusers must be referred for counseling to protect the fetus.

Box **5-4**   **Recognizing Potential Substances of Abuse**

Substance abusers and those who supply these substances constantly change the names and forms, but the substances are no less devastating whatever the name or form. Be aware of the most common drugs in your area and look for signs of abuse in your high-risk patients. Following is a brief alphabetical overview of some of the most commonly abused substances with the highest risk of addiction.

Alcohol (ETOH) is one of the most socially acceptable and most frequently abused drugs in our society. Alcohol depresses the central nervous system, causing loss of coordination, slurred speech, and double vision. In large amounts, alcohol depresses respiration and heart rate. Most states recognize blood alcohol content of greater than 0.10 as the legal definition of intoxication. Death by alcohol poisoning may result with blood alcohol levels over 0.40. Prolonged abuse of alcohol leads to alcoholism, malnutrition, cirrhosis of the liver, and death. Alcohol also has a devastating effect on a developing fetus.

Cocaine and crack cocaine are derived from the leaves of the coca plant but can be synthetically reproduced in laboratories. Both have strong stimulant effects on the central nervous system. Cocaine is used medically as a local anesthetic. Used properly in minor surgery, it deadens the local area and produces vasoconstriction to reduce bleeding at the site. As an addictive drug, it is ingested, rubbed on the mucous membranes, sniffed into the nose, or injected. Its euphoric effects last only about 30 minutes, meaning that the abuser needs frequent doses to maintain a "high." It is quickly and severely addicting, with multiple side effects such as hypertension, cardiac arrhythmias, seizures, respiratory arrest, and death. The crack form of cocaine is smoked, enters the cardiovascular system quickly, and can lead to cardiopulmonary collapse and death. All forms of cocaine cross the placental barrier and are very dangerous to the fetus.

Depressants, barbiturates, and tranquilizers depress the central nervous system. Used therapeutically, they reduce anxiety in certain stress disorders, prevent seizures, relieve insomnia, and aid in pain relief. Several forms are highly addictive. Patients who are not physically addicted frequently are so dependent on the effects of this class of drugs that they cannot function normally after withdrawal. Since their effects are depressive, abusers appear drowsy and lethargic, their speech is slurred, and their heart rate and blood pressure are low. Overdose leads to respiratory depression, coma, and death. They have many names, but are most commonly called "downers" or "tranqs."

Hallucinogens excite the central nervous system, causing hallucinations, mood changes, and delusions. They elevate all vital signs, including body temperature. LSD, PCP, mescaline, and peyote are all illegal, highly addicting hallucinogens. They have no medical use but may be used in strictly controlled psychiatric experiments. Abuse results in memory loss, seizures, coma, cardiopulmonary collapse, and death. Abusers may experience hallucinations for up to a year after withdrawal. Because reality and pain perception are so altered, abusers may injure themselves or others while under the influence. Signs of abuse vary with the hallucinogen, but most include agitation and loss of reality.

Marijuana is manufactured from the dried tops of the cannabis, or hemp, plant. Its many and constantly changing street names include "grass," "ganja," "pot," "weed," "joint," and "hashish." The product can be smoked or ingested. It produces euphoria and alters judgment, cognition, and sensory perception. Even low doses alter certain perceptions, depressing some, such as concentration and complex interpretations, and increasing or altering others,

Box **5-4**   **Recognizing Potential Substances of Abuse—Cont'd**

such as touch, taste, and smell. If mental illness is present in any form, the mind-altering chemicals increase the incidence of paranoia and schizophrenia. Signs of marijuana use include conjunctivitis, hunger, and either agitation or lethargy.

Narcotics are derived from the opium poppy or made synthetically in a laboratory. They alter sensory perception and produce euphoria. Medically, they are used to treat pain, suppress the cough reflex, constrict pupils, and decrease gastrointestinal motility in cases of nausea and vomiting. Included in this group are morphine, heroin, and meperidine (Demerol). Signs of abuse may include unconsciousness, stupor, decreased respirations, coma, and death.

Nicotine is highly addictive whether it is smoked or chewed. Along with alcohol, it is considered the most socially acceptable form of addiction and is a form of "slow motion suicide." Smokers are twice as likely as nonsmokers to develop cardiovascular disease. They have a greater risk of cancers of the lungs, mouth, throat, stomach, and bladder. Nicotine is physiologically addictive, which means that the reforming smoker suffers physiological withdrawal that includes insomnia, anxiety, and agitation. Stopping smoking cigarettes is extremely difficult and many smokers cannot do it alone. Social support groups can be very effective. Several new drugs have shown promise in breaking the addiction. They are available as patches, oral medications, and prescription gum.

Stimulants, such as amphetamine and its derivatives, excite the central nervous system to produce wakefulness and euphoria. The street names change frequently but include "black beauties," "pep pills," "ice," "uppers," and "speed." This group of drugs is used medically to treat narcolepsy, short-term fatigue, certain respiratory conditions, and depression. The many adverse effects include paranoia, hallucinations, and suicidal tendencies. Signs include those associated with stimulation such as agitation and increased heart rate and respirations.

As with any health care concern, it is better to prevent a problem than to treat it after it is firmly established. The following suggestions may help prevent abuse or addiction, or may make treatment more effective in relieving an established addiction.

- Help potential or at-risk patients deal with stress that leads to abuse. They need productive, not maladaptive, coping mechanisms. Substance abuse in addition to a stressful situation multiplies the problem; the stress is still there but is made worse by adding addiction.
- Help patients realize they can ask for help for anxiety, depression, or loneliness. With proper support, they should not need potentially addicting substances.
- Know the local names and forms of the drugs you may encounter. Almost all drugs are used over wide areas, but some are more common in certain populations than others, and the names change frequently.
- Learn to recognize the signs and symptoms of chronic abuse and overdose. With the variety and availability of destructive drugs, you may be the patient's first and best resource for assistance.
- Educate patients to talk with physicians regarding potentially addicting medications. Patients who we know or suspect are at risk for addiction should have other medication choices.

- Never moralize with addictive patients to make them feel guilty; they know it is wrong but are powerless to stop. They need help, not lectures. As always, talk with the physician about the patient and document your concerns.
- Watch for drug-seeking behaviors, such as patients who ask for specific controlled substances before trying other means to relieve symptoms. Patients who self-diagnose and self-prescribe may be at risk.
- Beware of clusters of patients asking for the same controlled substances. Many addictive drugs have great street value.
- Keep education brochures up-to-date and available. Know the support groups in your area to call quickly when necessary.
- Call for help if you are frightened by drug-related psychosis in a patient. Patients in drug-induced paranoia will not listen to reason. Do not put yourself in danger.
- Refer patients to support groups such as Alcoholics Anonymous or Narcotics Anonymous. Because abuse is so disruptive to families, urge caregivers and family members to join support groups such as Al-Anon or Alateen. Nicotine and smokers' support groups help those who cannot stop without social or psychological support. Some can stop abruptly; others need strong support.

Medications are so readily available and stress levels are so high in health care, that it may not be just patients whose substance abuse causes concern. Health care professionals are at high risk for addiction. If the abuser is the physician, notify the Impaired Physician Committee in your area. If the abuser is a coworker, report your concerns to a supervisor. Keep careful documentation and be very sure of the situation before making an accusation. However, you owe it to coworkers and patients to protect the profession from substance abuse.

The following signs should alert you to a problem in the work place:

- Watch for secretive behavior, moodiness, and hostility, particularly if it is out of character.
- Workers who always volunteer to control the medicine cabinet may be exhibiting drug-seeking behavior. No one person should be in charge of the narcotics supply in the health care setting. This should be a shared responsibility.
- Repeated absenteeism on Friday and Monday may be a sign of weekend substance abuse.
- Look for chronic conjunctivitis without accompanying allergies or infection.
- Chronic sore throat and a hoarse cough without other signs should be a red flag warning. These signs indicate a problem whether or not drugs are the cause.
- Chronic fatigue or agitation may indicate abuse. Abusers may alternate between periods of intense activity and periods of lethargy.

Substance abuse and addiction are problems in all cultures and socioeconomic groups; users cannot be stereotyped. Be alert to help potential and current abusers before they harm themselves or others with this destructive behavior.

UNDERSTANDING MEDICATION

Millions of dollars are spent annually in this country on illnesses caused by drugs prescribed to make us well. The U.S. Department of Health and Human Services (DHHS) estimates that roughly half of all prescription medications are taken improperly, sometimes with severe consequences. Because of the great potential for interaction and adverse reactions in medication administration, understanding how and when to take medications and why they were ordered can have a profound effect on recovery from illness or maintenance of an acceptable level of health.

Many sources are available to learn about the drugs prescribed in your facility. The Physician's Desk Reference (PDR), the U.S. Pharmacopoeia (USP), and several good, brief reference books outline the properties of most current medications. The National Council on Patient Information and Education (NCPIE), a nonprofit organization in Washington D.C. (666 Eleventh Street, N.W., Suite 810, Washington, DC 20001), will provide literature for you and your patients or will refer you to other sources for information. If certain medications are prescribed routinely in your facility, talk with the prescribing physicians about using these resources to create brief, understandable patient education material to supply with medications or prescriptions. Pharmacists are required to provide standard instructions with each prescription, but no patient is ever over-informed. Pharmaceutical representatives, or "drug reps," also may supply patient-friendly information written by the pharmaceutical company, but, like those supplied by pharmacists, they may not be appropriate for certain patient populations with low literacy levels. Tell your patients about the medication, ask for questions, and have a report-back system in place for later questions, but always supply patients with written, understandable patient education material (Box 5-5).

If it is your responsibility to educate patients regarding medication administration, such as inhaled, injected, transdermal, or oral, this specific detailed information will be covered in other courses in your program. Regardless of how medications are administered and

Box **5-5**   **Talking about Medicine**

Well-informed, proactive patients ask questions such as those listed below. Patients who do not know what to ask need your help to understand that they should be active participants in health care decisions. Answers to questions such as these may help.

- What is the name of this drug?
- Why am I taking it? What should it do for me? What should it not do for me?
- Is it available in a generic form? If it is not, is there another form available or another treatment option?
- How many times a day should I take it?
- Does it matter when or how I take it (early morning, late at night, empty stomach or with food)?
- Is there anything I should avoid while taking this medication, such as driving, sun exposure, or certain foods?
- How many pills, capsules, or spoonfuls should I take?
- Does it require special handling (refrigeration, dark cabinet)?
- Is it safe to take with my vitamins and minerals? My other medications? My usual diet?
- Have there been reports of unsafe interactions?
- If I miss a dose, should I double up or should I skip that dose and resume the schedule at the next dosage time? What harm might I expect if I cannot stick with the schedule?
- What side effects might I experience? Which ones should I report and to whom?
- How long will I be on this medication? One week, one month, or the rest of my life?
- Is it OK to have alcohol with this medication?
- Is it OK to stop this medication if I feel better before it is gone? Or if I feel worse? Should I report to you if I stop it?

whose responsibility it is to educate patients in their use, this is a whole team effort with evaluations of understanding made by everyone who interacts with the patient.

- Determine whether the patient is vision-impaired. Can he see the labels well enough to know which medication he is taking? Can he measure it? Can you provide him with visual aids to make measuring and administration easier?
- Does she have the manual dexterity to draw up medications and self-inject? Should she be referred to a home health service if there is no one available to help with administration?
- Can he understand which medication must be taken at what time and in what manner? Can the routine be simplified?
- Does she understand that over-the-counter (OTC) and so-called "natural" remedies may interact badly with prescription drugs? Can you help her see how dangerous mixing substances can be?
- Does he understand how important it is to take the medication as prescribed and what might happen if he does not follow the proper regimen?
- Should you demonstrate with special memory aids, such as divided dosage boxes to make remembering dosage times easier?

Since medical treatment usually continues beyond your involvement with the patient, helping patients and caregivers understand how medications affect health is as important as administering them yourself or explaining how they should be taken.

SAFETY FIRST

Safety and security are so important that they are included in Maslow's Hierarchy of Needs (see Chapter 4, "Educating Patients") just above the most basic physiological needs. Achieving other, higher goals must wait until safety is ensured. It is as important that we help patients understand how to remain safe as it is to help them maintain health. Although not technically an illness, traumatic injuries are as devastating to health as any disease or disorder, and, in many cases, are as avoidable with proper care. Injuries are one of the top five causes of premature death in our general population, after heart disease, stroke, cancer, and pulmonary disease. Since the top four causes of death are considered degenerative diseases and usually affect the older populations, preventing injuries or unsafe choices is especially important in maintaining the health of our younger patients.

The need for safety includes all ages, but certain groups are more likely to suffer specific types of injuries than others. Certain areas expose patients to injuries not present in other places, such as hypothermia in the North versus hyperthermia in the South, or a hay mowing accident on a farm versus a jellyfish sting at the beach. It is not within the scope of this text to address the safety issues in every conceivable situation but to urge all health care workers to be aware of safety concerns specific to their geographic area and patient populations.

Factors that affect safety and injury control include the following:

- Developmental life stages. Safety education should begin before conception with healthy choices for both parents and must continue throughout the pregnancy. The American Academy of Pediatrics provides age-appropriate Anticipatory Guidance information to all pediatricians to be supplied to parents during well-child checkups. For example, brochures present information regarding safe cribs, age-appropriate toys, approved and properly installed car seats, cabinet locks, and vigilant supervision. Information regarding the teen years is understandably directed at educating teens regarding risky behavior (see below).

Adult safety education involves cautioning patients about prudent lifestyle choices, avoiding potentially violent situations, and the increase in accidents caused by stress and exhaustion. Our elderly populations are more likely to suffer fall injuries as a side effect of medications or weakening sensory perception.

- Lifestyle choices. Risky sex, smoking, drinking, drug abuse, dangerous hobbies and sports, and a reduced perception of danger lead to many avoidable injuries. These risky behaviors are potentially dangerous to bystanders and other persons as well, as seen in drunk-driving accidents.
- Health status. Patients who are weak, frail, dizzy, or impaired or who have altered sensory perception are more likely to be injured than those who are in good health with good reflexes.
- Psychological status. Stress interferes with the perception of our surroundings, causing us to be too distracted to pay attention to potential danger. Depression, fatigue, and disorientation also reduce awareness and lead to accidents.
- Environment. Our homes and communities can be unsafe places. Many homes are unsafe, with poor lighting, clutter, hazardous material, unsanitary conditions, guns, and vicious dogs. Many areas of our country are considered unsafe, or may be safe for certain ages and not for others. For example, a farm with many implements may be safe for persons with proper judgment but not for small children who could be seriously injured.
- Occupation. The Office of Safety and Health Administration (OSHA) requires a safe workplace, but accidents still occur far too often. Loud noises, repetitive motion, dust, radiation, or chemical exposure and machinery without safeguards or proper worker training lead to many debilitating illnesses and injuries.
- High risk factors. Evaluate the safety awareness of patients and caregivers. For example, parents who always use approved safety seats for children and seat belts for themselves are probably compliant in other areas of health and safety also. Adults with dependent parents who always accompany the parent and are involved in appropriate decision-making usually safeguard elderly relatives in the home as well. Patients and caregivers who seem unaware of high-risk behaviors may need extra attention and vigilance.

Suggestions for helping patients and caregivers include the following:

- Check your facility from a safety perspective for workers and patients. Look at it through an older person's eyes and from a child's-eye viewpoint.
- Develop a fall prevention protocol for the agency. What can you do from the front door to the patient care area to make it safer?
- Provide safety pamphlets and brochures appropriate for your patient population.
- Help patients identify safety factors in their personal environment and lifestyle choices.
- Enlist the aid of your local fire and police departments to inspect the homes of patients at high risk. This is a valuable free public service that should not be overlooked in providing patient safety.
- Observe patterns of suspected falls, burns, or other injuries that might indicate impairment or other high-risk factors, including abuse.
- Be alert for medication side effects such as dizziness or weakness; look for recent changes in health, such as a debilitating illness or loss of sensory perception.
- Use every opportunity to reinforce safety education. For example, provide pediatric Anticipatory Guidance education for parents at each developmental stage of childhood, urge patients and caregivers to become involved with CPR training, and ensure that all patients understand medication side effects that could lead to falls.

INCORPORATING COMPLEMENTARY AND NONTRADITIONAL THERAPIES

Alternative and complementary treatments have a long and credible history but until recently have been disregarded by the medical community. To understand the difference, *alternative* therapy is used in place of traditional medicine, and *complementary* treatments are used in addition to traditional medicine. The science-oriented basis for current medicine has dismissed the ancient arts with their emphasis on touch and an absence of technology, even though we understand that many factors are involved in any healing process. If this were not true, we all would heal or recover at the same rate with the same treatment. Clearly, other factors must be considered. Even the traditional medical establishment recognizes that patients who believe they will improve generally do better than those who are convinced they will not. We know that placebos work many times, even for organic rather than simply psychosomatic pain. We know that touching patients with kindness and compassion measurably lowers stress levels. Knowing these concepts and that the patient's state of mind has much to do with recovery has led forward-thinking health care workers to consider that prevention, healing, and recovery may lie in treatments other than medications and surgery. Many physicians are now accepting alternative therapies and including certain complementary models in practice. For example, an orthopedist or a physician with a sports medicine practice may have a credentialed massage therapist or acupuncture or acupressure technician on staff as an adjunct or complement to more traditional medicine.

To understand how illness and healing are inseparably linked within us, remember that the mind and body are two parts of the whole person. What affects the body impacts the mind, and vice versa. For example, many of us have stress-induced headaches, and while it may work to medicate the pain, is it not better to relieve the cause than the effect? Much of alternative medicine works on this theory. Relieving the cause of the symptom is more likely to work than attacking the symptom and leaving the cause intact. Many organic illnesses have an emotional component, such as a stress-filled life leading to hypertension or gastric ulcers. The organic signs and symptoms can be relieved by medication or other treatment, but relieving or eliminating the precipitating stress is ultimately more beneficial.

Cultural diversity has led many traditional-minded health care workers to reconsider the ancient arts. If your patient expresses a belief in these therapies or is of an ethnic group with a strong spiritual background, use your most compassionate communication to determine whether a healer is involved in the patient's care. Many herbal preparations prescribed by natural healers interact badly with conventional medicine and may compromise recovery from illness or surgery. Certain practitioners rely solely on "natural" remedies that may be dangerous to the patient who would benefit from a combination of traditional and nontraditional therapy. Not everything that is "natural" is safe; consider how many poisonous "natural" leaves and berries have made their way into folk medicine. Know as much as you can about each type of alternative or complementary treatment and the evolving trends so that you can appropriately advise your patients. Most alternative and complementary therapies cause no additional problems but may delay diagnosis and treatment if used rather than standard therapy.

Never criticize your patients' choices, but urge them to discuss everything with the physician. The following suggestions may help you interact successfully with patients who choose to use a more holistic approach than our current medical practices.

- Since most nontraditional healers spend far more time with patients than current medical practice, take the hint and avoid making patients feel rushed. Spend as much quality time as is practical listening to and interacting with patients.
- Reinforce the physician's advice and alert the physician to the patient's questions regarding other therapies.
- If the patient feels that the current illness is voodoo or a hex, he will need the same type of healer to remove the source. If you react with disbelief or ridicule, you will immediately destroy any rapport you have established.
- Understand your dominant population's beliefs. Hispanics and Latinos may refer to a curandero, island people may consult root doctors, and others may be more comfortable with spiritualists. Each population has preferred herbs, beliefs, and rituals. Learn all that you can about the groups in your area.

Avoiding Quacks

Without the regulation of formal organizations such as the American Medical Association, certain alternative healing practices attract greedy con artists known as "quacks." They prey on patients who are uncomfortable with modern technology and its apparent lack of compassion. If a patient is displeased with the level of care he receives from his doctor, he may be more open to the confidence inspired by self-proclaimed healers. Patients frequently feel that a physician's technical knowledge is less important than the amount of quality time spent listening, explaining, touching, and relating to them. Most patients want and need to feel valued by their health care providers. In the absence of compassion in traditional medicine, the conning professions provide this service in abundance.

Caution your patients to watch for quacks who promise cures and who cannot produce verifiable, credible credentials. Remind them to use common sense: if it sounds too good to be true, it probably is. Unfortunately, the Internet has become the source of much misinformation and quackery. Help your patients sift through current printed and electronic information by watching for the following:

- If the cure is advertised in the back of a magazine, complete with testimonials, be very skeptical.
- If the medicine has secret ingredients known only to tribes in Third World countries, this is not a good choice.
- If the medication is available only by mail, be very cautious.
- If the information is found on the Internet, find out who sponsors the site. Information from sites endorsed by the American Medical Association, for example, is well researched and credible.
- Look for statements of ethics, advertising, and privacy. A seal of approval by an agency such as Health on the Net promises standards of reliability. Or look for verifiable standards such as the Health Web Site Accreditation Program (www.urac.org) established by The American Accreditation Health Care Commission.
- If the "cure" sounds miraculous, check it out in www.quackwatch.com. This site keeps up with health care frauds and myths.
- Check more than one site. Never rely on just one site for information through the Internet, no matter how reliable the source.

Constant vigilance for opportunities to educate our patients about ways to maintain or restore health is a challenge for the whole health care team. The reward for this challenge is a healthier, happier patient.

Taking the Chapter to Work

Now, let's meet Lynelle and see how she has applied this chapter information in the workplace.

Lynelle is working for an internist. She is caring for a 52-year-old woman who comes into the office with very vague complaints. The patient states that she "has no energy" and is having "trouble sleeping." Lynelle looks at the medical record and sees that she has been a patient for 15 years and has no previous medical problems. Lynelle also sees that the patient is an executive secretary for a prestigious law firm. As Lynelle takes her blood pressure she notices that the patient is dressed in dirty clothes and that her hair has not been combed. Lynelle asks the patient if she went to work today. The patient states that she "called in sick to work." Lynelle followed that response by asking the patient about work absenteeism. The patient states that "she doesn't care about work or her friends." The patient then explains that "her last child has gone off to college and that she is very lonely and sad." Lynelle communicates these observations and facts to the physician. The physician sees the patient and makes a diagnosis of depression. Lynelle's excellent communication and observation skills played an important role in helping this patient.

Beyond the Classroom Exercises

Your Assignment Board

The following exercises will help you apply what you learned in the chapter. Place a check beside the assignments your instructor has given you. When you have completed the assignment, place a check in the completed column.

		Assigned	*Completed*
Checking Your Comprehension	(Textbook)	❑	❑
Expanding Critical Thinking	(Textbook)	❑	❑
Communication Surfer Exercises	(Textbook and Internet)	❑	❑
Communication Tree Branch #7	(CD-ROM)	❑	❑
Communication Tree Branch #8	(CD-ROM)	❑	❑
Voice Mail Message #5	(CD-ROM)	❑	❑

Checking Your Comprehension

Write a brief answer for each of the following assignments.
1. Name six factors that can affect holistic health.
2. Describe five diets that physicians commonly order for recovering patients.
3. Describe five types of vegetarian diets.
4. Compare isokinetic, isometric, and isotonic exercises.
5. List eight signs and symptoms a patient may experience if stress is not relieved.
6. List nine coping mechanisms commonly seen in the health care setting.
7. Describe eight common addictive substances.
8. List six questions that would be important to discuss with patients regarding their medications.
9. Explain six factors that can affect the safety and injury rate of patients.

Expanding Critical Thinking

1. Think in terms of quality of life reflected in the following diseases and disorders. In your opinion, list them in order of negative impact on a person's life. Outline ways the quality of life is diminished. Which do you think would be most difficult to control?
   a. Addiction to controlled substances
   b. Addiction to tobacco
   c. Addiction to alcohol
   d. Obesity
   e. Heart disease
   f. Type 2 or insulin-dependent diabetes mellitus
   g. Hypertension
2. Look again at the problems listed above. Which ones do you think earn the patient more sympathy? Why do you think this is so? Which ones earn the patient more negative reaction? Why?
3. What do you think would be the most difficult health habit to form? Which would be most beneficial? How hard are you willing to work to achieve this habit?
4. How do you think stress factors have changed since your parents were your age? Your grandparents? How do you think these factors will change for your children?
5. How do you think achieving your career goals will affect your stress factors? Will your stress levels improve, get worse, or simply change to other factors?
6. If it is true that many small hassles are as hard to handle as a major stressor, make a list of the small, noncritical but annoying things that happen to you in the course of a day. If these small occurrences will always happen, how might you change your response to each to make them less bothersome? Explain how these small stressors could affect someone already coping with illness.
7. If drugs were available to improve your quality of life, but would shorten your life by a number of years, how many years would you give up for the following?
   a. Physical strength
   b. Perfect health
   c. Genius intelligence
   d. Great popularity
   e. Prodigious talent
   f. Movie star or model appearance
8. Does it matter to you how much alcohol people drink? How many drinks would it take to make you uncomfortable for the following people:
   a. Your pregnant friend
   b. Your parents
   c. Your date or spouse
   d. Your supervisor or employer physician
   e. Your pastor or other religious leader
   f. Yourself

Continued

Expanding Critical Thinking—Cont'd

9. Keep a food diary for a full 48 hours. Register your calories, fat grams, and carbohydrates. From the Internet, print a USDA food guide pyramid appropriate for your age and ethnicity. Have you included foods from all groups on the USDA pyramid in the recommended amounts? If your diet did not follow the guidelines, keep another record for the next 48 hours and try to stay within the recommendations for a prudent diet. How hard was it to stay within the guidelines? What do you think your chances are for making these changes permanent?

10. To better understand the interaction of medications and supplements, choose two popular medications, or medications that you take, and research the interaction with vitamin and mineral preparations or popular herbal supplements.

11. Look back over the stress response under the section in the chapter called "The Stress Factor" and for each response listed, explain how this natural reaction over time can lead to many of the stress-related illnesses that plague our patients. For example, over time, how do you think an increase in the normal heart rate, blood glucose levels, respiratory rates, and so forth, will affect our patients' long-term health?

12. You have battled weight for years with varying degrees of success. Today you are caring for a 16-year-old girl diagnosed with anorexia nervosa who is in for dehydration and malnutrition. She states, "I won't take those vitamins the doctor ordered, they will make me fat." How will you respond?

13. Refer to the Food Guide Pyramids on the Internet. Plan a 1-day diet for the following people.
    a. A 4-year-old boy
    b. A 16-year-old vegetarian girl
    c. A 75-year-old woman with osteoporosis
    d. A 40-year-old overweight man
    e. Yourself

14. Should a person contemplating suicide be institutionalized or restrained "for his own good"? Explain your answer.

15. Do you think suicide is a crime, a sin, or a personal option? Are there any circumstances conceivable under which suicide is justifiable?

16. Have you ever been tempted to end your life? What were the circumstances? What helped you change your mind?

17. Look through your home for safety factors. Kneel at a child's level for a child's-eye view. Put on smudged or dark glasses for an older person's perspective of the safety of your home. Make a list of the hazards you find and what you can do to correct them. Call your local fire department and ask for a home fire inspection. Call your local police department and ask for a home safety inspection. Bring the forms to class with you for discussion.

Communication Surfer Exercises

1. Go to a search engine and find the United States Department of Agriculture (USDA) Food Guide Pyramids. Print the information listed for diets recommended for the general public, for the elderly, for children, and for at least two ethnic groups. Compare the pyramids. List ways they are alike and ways they are different.

2. Using a search engine, find the National Dairy Council's (NDC) nutritional guidelines. How are they different from the USDA Food Guide Pyramids? Do you think they are easier to work with or harder? Print the guidelines and create a patient teaching guide explaining to patients how to stay within the recommendations.

3. Assume a patient asked you for information about the benefits of yoga versus Pilates. Using a search engine, find at least six sites that have information on yoga and Pilates. Create a list of the benefits of each type of exercise.

4. Stress can lead to many health problems. Find 10 sites that have valuable information about managing stress. Create a list of stress reduction techniques. How can you communicate this information to your patients?

5. Go to a search engine and find four sites that provide information regarding depression. Create a list of 10 ways to promote communication with a depressed patient.

6. Using a search engine, find five fad diet sites. Using the information from these sites, how could you communicate the risks and benefits associated with each diet?

7. Find the National Diabetes Association website. What information does this site communicate to patients with diabetes? Does it communicate the information in an effective format? Why or why not?

8. Using a search engine, find eight different types of support groups that are available in your area. Which support group site is best at communicating its purpose and resources?

9. Go to www.quackwatch.com. How would you describe this site to a patient? What are the benefits to teaching patients about this site?

6

COMMUNICATING THROUGH THE GRIEF PROCESS: WHEN WORDS ARE NOT ENOUGH

LEARNING OBJECTIVES

Upon successfully completing this chapter, you will be able to:

- Describe the changing professional views in the discussion of dying and death.
- List and explain Engel's stages of grief.
- List and explain Kübler-Ross's stages of grief.
- Describe how spiritual beliefs affect the grief experience.
- Explain cultural concepts of death and methods of displaying grief.
- Explain how views of dying and death change through the life span.
- Identify ways to protect yourself from "burnout" when coping with grieving patients.
- Give examples of support groups for the grieving patient or caregiver.

KEY TERMS

Anticipatory grief	Euthanasia	Thanatology
Bereaved, bereavement	Mourning	
Euphemism	Palliative	

Test Your Communication **IQ**

Before reading this chapter, complete this short self-assessment test. Decide which statements are true and which are false.

1. Bereavement is the first step in the grieving process and should last no more than 1 month.
2. It is important to focus your communication more on the patient than on the caregivers' needs.
3. During an illness crisis, a patient's religious faith always becomes deeper and more solid.
4. A statement such as "Grandma passed away during her sleep" is comforting and reassuring to a young child.
5. A statement such as "I know how you are feeling right now" is comforting to a patient who has been newly diagnosed with a terminal illness.
6. Patients with terminal illnesses should always be encouraged to attend support groups to discuss their feelings and fears about death.
7. Dr. Elisabeth Kübler-Ross identified the various stages of death or loss and promoted public awareness of this topic.

Results

Statement number seven is true; all other statements are false. How did you do? Read the chapter to find more information on these topics.

Until the middle of this past century, most people died at home by their mid-50s with very little medical intervention and no technological life support. Death was usually the result of accidents or acute contagious or infectious diseases; there was little that medicine could do to keep people alive for very long. Families kept their dead at home until burial, which was usually in a private family graveyard or the local church cemetery. Burying the dead nearby kept them as close as possible to their family and allowed the family to visit and continue the relationship after death. The rituals and public displays of **mourning** (the outward display of grief) and the support of close communities comforted survivors. Most families were large and extended so that everyone experienced the death of family members as a natural part of life.

As medical technology advanced and antibiotics cured many of the infectious illnesses that killed our ancestors, the median age for death extended to the late 70s and is still rising. Care of the dying, usually from chronic degenerative diseases, is now the responsibility of hospitals, not families. Mortuaries handle our dead and bury them away from us in generic public cemeteries. Many people no longer see death as part of life but as something to be avoided at all costs, even if those costs are quantity of days versus quality of life. In many cases, the emphasis is on extending life by every possible medical and technological advantage. The definition of death has changed from simply "an absence of life" and is measured by complex technological means such as cerebral and brainstem function. Hearts are restarted, pulmonary function is maintained, and organs are transplanted; dying takes longer and is increasingly complex. Some feel that we are prolonging dying, rather than prolonging life. This has led to a backlash of moral and ethical dilemmas that include assisted suicide, do not resuscitate (DNR) orders, "comfort measures only" (no life support measures), and "terminal weaning" (slowly removing mechanical life support as death is inevitable). **Euthanasia**, literally "good death," has been divided into concepts of allowing the terminally ill to die without intervention versus assisting them to die by removing all life support. The question of how to define the end of life is no longer simply a medical decision; it is a strong political and religious issue.

The public is beginning to see that while saving lives is a noble purpose, prolonging life without quality is a questionable achievement that may need to be considered on a case-by-case basis. This text will not attempt to address ethical, legal, and moral issues but will concentrate on understanding and communicating with those experiencing great loss and those responsible for their care. Remember, too, that in the medical setting, great loss may involve degrees of illness and may not necessarily mean that death is imminent. Your personal involvement in dying and death will depend on your specialty and your career choice, but dealing with the loss of health is common to almost all areas of medicine. The mechanics of death as it pertains to your specialty will be covered in other areas of your course work.

WORKING THROUGH GRIEF, LOSS, AND BEREAVEMENT

Grief is deep mental anguish caused by the actual or perceived (imagined) loss of anything we value. An actual loss is apparent to others, such as the death of a loved one, a divorce, or loss of a job. Perceived loss is apparent only to the one suffering the loss and may include intangible concepts, such as loss of self-esteem or failure to reach personal goals. Actual or perceived losses include life (yours, a significant other's, or a well-loved pet's), health, a relationship, security, your home, belongings, a job, or your value to society. We cope with small losses, or "deaths," all through our lives: when we grow up and lose our youth, move from place to place, separate from friends and family, even when we lose valued objects. All of these losses help prepare us for the ultimate loss, which, of course, is death. Grief is the price we pay for caring for someone or something, and through the process of grief, we learn to accept the reality of loss. The intensity and duration of the grief process is proportional to the value we place on the loss; therefore, grief is experienced, in many cases, just as acutely for loss of good health as for an actual death.

Terms used to describe the process of coping with loss vary through the psychological community. Some authorities use terms such as mourning and **bereavement** interchangeably; others insist that they describe different concepts. We, the authors, have chosen to use the most commonly accepted definitions for terms such as *bereaved* to signify a person experiencing bereavement, the state of deep grief or loss. *Mourning* is the period of accepting the loss. This period is very personal, and the behaviors and rituals in its outward display are determined by our culture, which we will cover later in this chapter. Grief is generally thought to be an inward expression and mourning is described as more likely obvious to others.

Coping with loss may begin when patients or family members learn of the terminal or life-changing nature of an illness. If there is time to prepare for the loss, and grief can begin early, this is called **anticipatory grief**. Patients and families may have years, months, or days, or the loss may be instant. Anticipatory grief either by the sick or dying or by those who care for them may disrupt emotional connections as each person prepares for the loss or the change in family dynamics. During this time, communication is difficult but must be maintained to nurture relationships as long as possible. If grief begins with the loss of a loved one through death with no warning, as in sudden or accidental death, or the sudden loss of a body part or personal health, there is no time to prepare. Emotional forces and thought processes are scattered as the shock of loss overwhelms physical and mental defenses. There is no time to gather the coping mechanisms that protect us from emotional overload. Grief from a sudden, violent death frequently is more acute than for death allowing for anticipatory grief and preparation. Grief is just as heartfelt no matter how it is presented, but it may be easier to withstand by having the process spread over a manageable time period.

Since everyone experiences grief at some time, our minds have adapted by developing means of adjusting to loss. Review coping mechanisms in Chapter 5, "Communicating Wellness," to understand how these work to protect us from overload. The initial physical response to grief usually includes panic, difficulty swallowing, increased heart rate and blood pressure, exhaustion, insomnia, muscle pain, altered eating patterns, and headaches. Sadness and depression significantly lower resistance to opportunistic diseases, which may lead to physical illness in addition to emotional stress. These are the types of symptoms patients and family members bring to health care workers when they become overwhelming and are a sign that coping mechanisms are not working. Our responsibility as health care workers involves offering our strength to patients and caregivers as they learn to cope with grief (Fig. 6-1).

Theories on Dealing with Loss

When doctors had little in their black bags to actually save patients from death or disease, doctors, patients, and families seemed more willing to accept that death or disability was inevitable. As medical technology extended life by decades, death and disability were no

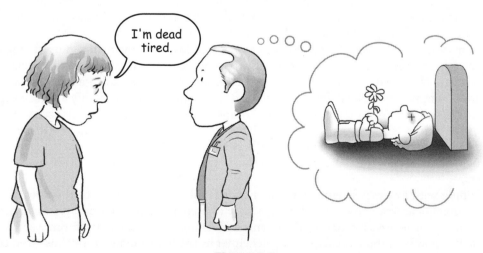

Figure 6-1

longer seen as acceptable options, and the subjects were no longer discussed. Everyone involved during much of the 1900s felt that to acknowledge death, or even loss of an acceptable health status, was to admit defeat. Physicians rarely discussed death, and many felt it was a personal failure on their part if a patient died—a failure of both medical technology and the doctor's proficiency. This is hard to understand, since we currently encourage open communication and patient empowerment. Some physicians still feel that to discuss death with the patient and family implies that the physician is giving up. Although the majority of patients and families want to know if death is close, or if healing is not probable, many health care professionals prefer not to acknowledge even the possibility. Not admitting that loss is near sends conflicting, or incongruent, cues of "everything is fine" and nonverbal cues that it definitely is not. Puzzled patients may think, "Your words say I am OK, but your expression says I am not."

Since the subject cannot be avoided, the backlash against secrecy, denial, and evasion is growing. **Thanatology**, the study of dying and death, is as old as the practice of medicine, but its credibility as a separate topic is fairly recent. As long ago as 1895, Sigmund Freud (1856-1939), an Austrian neurologist, wrote about the subject in "Mourning and Melancholia" and cautioned that grief and loss should be faced and worked through to avoid long-term depression. For many years, most articles and discussions on the subject were written for the health care or mental health professions and were not available to the general public.

G. L. Engel was one of the first medical writers to address dying and death in a manner that those outside of the medical profession could understand. In an article for the *American Journal of Nursing* in 1964 entitled "Grief and Grieving," Engel divided the grief process along these lines:

- Shock/disbelief: The "not me" stage. Patients withdraw from both physical and emotional contact and experience physical symptoms of stress or depression. Disbelief may have the benefit of delaying grief until the patient or family is better able to respond to the loss. Early disbelief and denial may be healthier and easier to manage than the panic many people experience when trying to process the shock too quickly.
- Developing awareness: The "why me" stage. Guilt and anger are normal during this phase. Guilt is more apparent if the loss was brought on by high-risk behavior or imprudent choices. Anger may be directed outward if the cause was an accident or violence.
- Restitution: This stage involves the "leave-taking" rituals surrounding loss (funerals, wakes, and so forth). Rituals give us comforting established cultural steps to follow when it is hard to make independent decisions. We know through our rituals what our society expects of us. In conservative cultures, there are usually clearly defined times and behaviors for each stage and step, such as how long to wear black as a sign of mourning, or when it is acceptable to remarry.
- Resolving the loss: coping with the feeling of loss. The bereaved describe themselves as "hollow" or "empty." Depression is common in this step. Watch for ways to help the grieving through this difficult time.
- Idealization: Concentrating on the worth of the loss. Persons in this stage will not look realistically at what was lost and will not tolerate negative thoughts or discussions regarding the loss. Many hoard possessions and reminders of whatever or whomever they have lost. For example, an athlete who is now a paraplegic will not part with sports equipment, or a widow may keep her husband's clothes for years.

- Acknowledgement or outcome: This final stage allows for realistic planning, saying good-bye, and tying up loose ends as the need to dwell on the loss becomes less overwhelming.

During this same time of developing public awareness of the topic of death, two prominent sociologists, Barney Glaser and Anselm Strauss, wrote "Awareness of Dying" in 1965 and "Time for Dying" in 1968. They outlined a series of steps or stages common to most issues of loss, which included shock, partial denial, denial, preparatory grief, hope, and letting go. These steps were very much like those described by Engel, and later by Dr. Elisabeth Kübler-Ross (see below). Glaser and Strauss, and others who wrote at this time regarding loss, seemed focused not so much on death as on receiving catastrophic news. Their theory seems true, as we will see when patients are told they have a debilitating or life-changing disease or disorder, whether or not it is life-threatening.

Dr. Elisabeth Kübler-Ross, a Swiss-born American psychiatrist, brought the discussion into the open and made the general public aware of the debate. Dr. Kübler-Ross wrote extensively on grief, including "On Death and Dying" in 1969, "Questions and Answers on Death and Dying" in 1974, and "Living with Death and Dying" in 1981, among others. Dr. Kübler-Ross wrote her articles on a level that the public could understand and made us aware that death and loss are stages of life to be worked through, and that open discussion helps everyone to cope with this unavoidable issue.

Although there are many detractors and philosophical disagreements about Dr. Kübler-Ross's theories, the steps or stages she outlined include the following.

- Denial, refusing to accept the loss: Expect statements such as, "No, this can't be!" "You are wrong!" "Those are not my test results!" Patients may ask for more tests, second opinions, more surgery. Survivors may demand or refuse to see the deceased, hoping that if they refuse to believe what they see and hear that this loss will not be true.
- Anger at everyone and everything: "Why did you let this happen to me?" "Why me?" Anger may be directed at the physician, at caregivers and loved ones, or at a Supreme Being. In many cases, anger is directed inward if the loss was caused by imprudent choices. Anger may become hostility as the griever withdraws from others who are not grieving and thinks, "How dare they be happy when I am so sad." Patients or caregivers in this step may refuse your compassion; however, remain available for comfort when you sense they may need you.
- Bargaining, trying to delay or avoid the inevitable: The bereaved may think, "If I follow the treatment plan, maybe I will get better." "If I pray hard enough, maybe it will go away." "Please let me live until June." (Note: Even if death is near in the first three stages, patients probably will prefer not to sign a DNR order or participate in a "Living Will.")
- Depression, the feeling of sadness, loneliness, or despair that accompanies loss: Continue to reach out during the depression stage; some patients need to talk and others prefer to retreat. Patients and survivors have a right to be depressed; denying them this step may disrupt the process. Be available for their needs. Remember the physiological effects of depression and be alert for ways to relieve the signs and symptoms.
- Acceptance, recognizing the inevitability of the loss: Persons in this stage begin to put their affairs in order. For the dying patient, the outside world begins to lose its meaning. These patients may be very self-centered as they reserve their remaining days. They are disengaging emotionally from the world and may prefer to have only one or two close relations around; some even exclude those they love. Peace and acceptance are more likely if the patient looks at the past with satisfaction, if goals have been met, and if resources are adequate for the final days and for the survivors. Survivors in the acceptance stage begin to make realistic plans for the coming changes.

Controversy still surrounds Kübler-Ross's work, but authorities in thanatology agree that she opened the discussion about death and grief that was desperately needed.

Each person experiences the stages of grief over varying lengths of time spent in each phase. There is no particular sequence from one step or stage to another. There are also frequent regressions to stages already experienced. Some stages are passed through quickly or not at all. For example, persons who are grieving may progress through denial and anger to bargaining, then back again to anger before progressing to other stages. Time spent in the stages or steps is intensely personal and inconsistent and cannot be hurried. Do not try to force bereavement into a generic formula and do not psychoanalyze the patient's or family's responses.

Most authorities agree that how we cope with stress throughout life helps predict how we will cope with grief. Coping mechanisms are covered in Chapter 5, "Communicating Wellness," but for our purposes we can presume that someone who has coped by denial all of his or her life will now spend most of the grieving time in denial. The person who reacts with anger to any frustration will become enraged at this thing so beyond personal control. Likewise, someone who is easily depressed may remain in the depression stage without progressing beyond that stage. Much depends also on how many other stressors are being juggled at the same time. For example, will money be a major problem, or will the needs of the survivors be covered? Will a parent be left with young children to rear alone? Is an adult child left with a complicated estate and many debts? If loose ends are tied up and realistic plans have been made, grief usually progresses more smoothly.

Age is also an important factor, as we will see later in this chapter. With life-long experiences with loss, the elderly usually progress to acceptance more quickly than children or young adults.

In the examples above, the focus is generally on the ill or dying patient; remember that the family and survivors are experiencing many of the same stages. Remember the caregivers as you administer to patients. The grief process is equally intense for those who are deeply affected by the loss. Family members are burdened with the care of the dying patient, or one whose health is compromised if this is not a terminal illness, and with changing family dynamics (Box 6-1). There may be a loss of security, great financial and physical burdens, added responsibility, and major life changes to accommodate the patient's care, particularly if the situation involves a long, debilitating illness. Although some patients and families fight

Box **6-1**   **TEARS**

With an emphasis on survivors of grief, both patients and family, professional grief workers use an acronym for bereavement that acknowledges the emotional release of tears, and the work that remains at the completion of Kübler-Ross's stages. The acronym TEAR is defined as follows.

T - To accept the reality of loss.

E - Experience the pain of loss.

A - Adjust to the loss.

R - Reinvest in a new reality.

Note that acceptance, the last stage outlined by Kübler-Ross, is the first step recognized by those working with survivors. Accepting loss begins the process of healing for the survivors of grief.

death to the last breath, in other cases, death may be a release and a relief for patients and caregivers.

The reason for the loss is also important in the process, whether the loss is life, health, security, or the like. Grief is easier if the loss is seen as honorable, such as paralysis after a heroic rescue, incapacity from burns suffered saving someone from fire, death in the pursuit of justice or excellence. Contrast those concepts to loss due to social vices—smoking, drinking, and unsafe sex. For example, death by suicide leaves survivors with many emotions different from death by other means. Survivors wonder why they did not see or recognize the signs and what they could have done differently to prevent the suicide. Guilt and shame are frequently complicating factors in socially unacceptable causes of grief.

A new factor in grief involves the acquired immune deficiency syndrome (AIDS) epidemic. Added to the normal progression of bereavement is the shame sometimes still associated with this disease. Regardless of the method by which patients were exposed to HIV, they and their caregivers frequently experience isolation and social rejection, removing them from the usual support systems available to other grieving persons. Partners of AIDS patients may not be accepted by the family of the dying patient and may not be allowed to grieve with other mourners, which denies them an important source of comfort. Even now, with more acceptance and understanding, patients still may die alone in isolation units, with very little personal contact and with no one to touch them for comfort.

We are mandated by our choice of profession to care for everyone who needs our skill and knowledge. We will cope with many infectious diseases, as well as diseases that could have been avoided by prudent choices; how these diseases were contracted should not concern us, the health and well-being of our patients in the present is our primary concern. Whatever your personal moral convictions, all patients must be treated with compassion and respect. Never in any manner display a behavior that may be interpreted as rejection to patients or caregivers. The cause of loss and the method of grieving cannot be considered in offering comfort and compassion. The grief process requires a therapeutic response whatever its form or cause.

When the pain of loss is accepted, healing begins. If the loss is not in death but in health and mobility, new skills must be learned, new roles assumed, and new life directions determined. If the loss is in death, the same adjustments are required of the survivors. Although waves of grief return at times, and for some people grief never goes away, survivors eventually begin to feel hope and joy again without the intense feeling of loss and emptiness.

The Importance of Spirituality

After the shock, disbelief, and anger of great loss, many patients and caregivers need spiritual assistance as much as they need medical attention. To communicate effectively, you need to understand a wide variety of spiritual needs. Rather than defining and outlining each religion's focus on death, we suggest that you study the predominant beliefs in your area that are different from your own; then expand your research to include other religions not represented locally. Knowing about other religious beliefs should not threaten your own beliefs but should broaden your acceptance of different cultures, which is vital to effective understanding and communication.

The spiritual beliefs you will encounter range from atheism (denial of a Supreme Being) through agnosticism (the belief that the existence of a Supreme Being is unknown and unknowable) to theism (the belief that the Supreme Being is real and personally involved in the lives of humans). Even theism ranges through many denominations, interpretations, and beliefs. All religions were established to reflect and focus beliefs in the purpose of being and the meaning of life. Most people seem to need to believe that life continues after death. Many early cultures buried possessions, even food, for the dead to use in the afterlife, and we still choose the most beautiful caskets and headstones that we can afford and dress our dead in their best clothes. Early Egyptian mummification was an attempt to overcome the decay of death, while today we embalm bodies and are experimenting with cryonics (therapeutic freezing), as advocates hope to thaw the deceased when cures are discovered for current diseases. However we may feel now, most early cultures felt that the afterlife was filled with peace and harmony after a difficult life on earth, although most religions have always believed in a place of eternal torment for those they felt deserved it. The belief in a benevolent afterlife is common to most established religions and is a strong component in acceptance of loss by death.

Our religious preference helps us decide how to cope with dying, death, and nonbeing, since all religions address end-of-life issues and immortality. It is easier for us to consider a world that existed without us before we were born than it is to think of life and eternity going on without us now. Our individual acceptance of death as the end of existence or the beginning of life eternal is based on beliefs certain religions find most comforting. Our religious beliefs help us determine answers to questions such as: Is death a transition phase to another life or an end of being? Are we going to a vengeful or a loving God? Will there be eternal punishment for sins and vices, or a reward for a life well lived? Answers to these and other questions about life and death are found in the stated beliefs of all religions.

Spiritual beliefs take on new and stronger meanings when our concepts of "being" are challenged. The crisis of illness may either shake or deepen faith as it brings about great change. Many people believe that if their faith is strong enough, there will be no suffering or death; when suffering continues or death occurs, it tests even strong faith. Well-meaning friends and family may urge patients and family members to pray harder, have more faith, believe more strongly; then if healing does not occur, everyone involved is likely to believe that faith was not strong enough to bring about a cure. Health care professionals know that miraculous, unexplainable cures happen every day in medicine, but that is why they are remarkable and why they are miracles, and why they sometimes do not happen. Be prepared for even deeper grief reactions if faith is shaken in the midst of the grief process.

From a practical standpoint, spiritual beliefs frequently affect medical practice. Patients and families come to us with strong beliefs about the right to life versus the right to die. Patients may refuse blood transfusions even if death is probable without replacing blood loss. They may demand or reject surgery. If it is within the law, families may refuse an autopsy for a deceased member. All of these issues are magnified if some family members believe one way and others believe differently.

Fortunately, as health care professionals, we do not make choices for our patients or families, but we have to live with the decisions made by others that may be the complete opposite of our beliefs. Even when this is true, we cannot impose what we believe on our patients or their families. However you may feel about dying, death, suffering and loss, and however much you may want to guide the bereaved to your view of spirituality, you must never impose your beliefs on patients or family members who would prefer that you did not. Introducing conflicting beliefs at this time is not appropriate. Watch for cues during this difficult and fragile time and retreat if your attempts at spiritual comfort increase stress rather than relieve the situation. Never in any manner communicate rejection of another's religious beliefs. If your faith demands that you share your beliefs with others, there are more appropriate times than during the grief process.

We may still witness to our faith without imposing our beliefs or bringing into question anyone else's interpretation of spirituality. For example, there is no reason you cannot offer to contact a chaplain or the patient's or family's spiritual advisor. With patients' or families' approval, having such a person near frees us to attend to physical needs, while those more appropriately trained offer spiritual comfort.

What must we do to ensure that spiritual needs are met during the grief process?

- Respect and learn about a variety of faiths and believe that each is as important to its members as yours is to you.
- Allow time alone with the spiritual leader and work around those who are grieving without intruding. Remain available to tend to physical needs as necessary.
- Never by any communication cues, verbal or nonverbal, imply that you question someone else's beliefs. This is not the time or place to debate religious issues.

Respecting someone else's religious beliefs should not challenge your spirituality. Recognizing everyone's freedom to worship, or not worship, is one of our most basic rights and is never more important than during the crisis of bereavement. Communicate your acceptance of differences and minister to the patient's physical needs.

CULTURAL PERSPECTIVES OF DYING AND DEATH

You will see as you work in medicine that some fatal or debilitating illnesses are more specific to certain groups than others. For example, hypertension leading to disability or death is more common among African-Americans than Asian-Americans. Poor people die of more correctable diseases at an earlier age and have higher infant mortality than rich people. Wealthy patients generally die of degenerative diseases later in life than disadvantaged patients. Certain other cultures place as much emphasis on shaman, curandera, or root doctors as they do on modern medicine and may turn to organized health care only as a last resort. All of these factors and many more affect how cultures view death and how they grieve. As we noted in Chapter 2, "Challenges to Communication," learning as much as you can about other cultures helps to communicate in every area of medicine, including dying and death.

Cultural perspectives of death are hard to discuss without also including religions common to different ethnic groups. Within each cultural group are also religious differences; for example, the white Protestant population covers so many broad groups that one belief, one mourning ritual, one view of dying and death would be impossible to define. The same is true of the Asian groups, the African-American population, or Hispanic-Americans. As we noted earlier regarding cultural challenges, there is rarely a consensus of beliefs even among friends and families, which leaves us with only broad generalizations for cultural views of dying, death, and grief. Among each group are rich and poor, educated and uneducated, as well as those who have assimilated into American culture and those who cling to ethnic traditions. For example, wealthy urban African-Americans may practice mourning rituals more like those of their white neighbors than those of poor African-American families. Conversely, poor whites may mourn more like poor African-Americans that they do like wealthy whites. To assign specific beliefs and characteristics to any group can slip easily into stereotyping (Box 6-2).

Cultures practice different mourning rituals and traditions that are comfortable to members of the group. For public display, we will see black arm bands, flags at half mast, wreaths signifying the continuous circle of life and days set aside to honor the dead, such as Presidents' Day, Memorial Day, and Martin Luther King Day. In North America, we usually prefer to honor our dead with funerals, flowers, eulogies (literally meaning "good words") and relatively restrained mourning. Although grief is personal, mourning is frequently for show and cannot be objectively measured. Some cultures are very vocal and demonstrative in mourning, weeping loudly and tearing at their clothes; others mourn silently; and still others celebrate death with joyful singing and dancing. Those who weep loudly probably do not feel grief any more deeply than those who were taught to display only discreet emotion. The restrained North American mourning displays must seem cold and unfeeling to cultures

Box **6-2**   **Cultural Demonstrations of Grief**

Broad generalizations regarding cultural beliefs and traditions are unavoidable; however, most sources support the following observations.

- African-Americans as a group are more demonstrative in grief than whites. Their religious beliefs include all denominations. However, their basic spirituality is grounded in the circle of life and death concept. Many early tribes felt that as long as someone was remembered and his name called at gatherings, that person still existed and entered the afterlife only when no one in the tribe remembered his name. This is a common tradition in many cultures, even the general white population, and is the basis for carrying on family given names (first or second names rather than the last name).
- Hispanic-Americans are of Mexican, Puerto Rican, or Cuban ancestry. They form stronger family ties than most whites and frequently live in extended family units, as other immigrant groups did in earlier eras. This may reflect a "safety in numbers" that whites and African-Americans no longer need. Hispanic-Americans are generally Catholic. Depending on ethnicity, some groups are more vocal in mourning than others. Mexican-Americans, and many other predominantly Catholic groups, observe November 2 as the "Day of the Dead" for the deceased to return to earth to visit with relatives.
- Asian populations may be Chinese, Filipino, or Japanese, among others. Asian-Americans are generally very restrained in mourning. This may be incorrectly interpreted as lack of emotion. They believe strongly in a benevolent afterlife. As the populations have adapted to American cultures, religious beliefs have expanded, but many remain Buddhists, Confuscians, and members of other Eastern-based religions. They are very accepting of death as necessary for rebirth, believing that each soul is reborn many times.
- Native-Americans have so assimilated with other dominant cultures that only broad generalizations can be made about mourning practices. Most believe in the cycle of life concept and see death as a natural part of life. Within the wide range of tribal customs, however, some tribes fear death and have extensive rituals for removing the "pollution" of death, while other tribes are less fearful in the presence of death. Some Native-American cultures still practice nature-based beliefs; others have adopted other forms of religion.

that show respect for the dead by obvious and dramatic behavior. All of these mourning rituals help the living pay tribute to the dead and usually are determined by our social customs or religion.

GRIEF AND LOSS ACROSS THE LIFESPAN

Our perceptions of loss change as we mature and can see beyond the immediate impact of grief. Obviously, adults understand loss better than young children, and the older the child is, the better he or she should be at recognizing that loss is an inevitable part of life. Older adults usually have experienced many losses and cope with end-of-life issues better than active, involved young adults or children of any age. As with different cultures and religions, individuals within each age group have many different coping skills, making it difficult to predict how any age will respond to grief and loss (see the Legal Eagle box).

Helping Children Cope with Loss

Responsible, loving parents would suffer harm or injuries or die themselves to protect their children from danger or illness. We are supposed to protect our children and feel powerless when we cannot. We immunize our children against illness, install child-proof cabinet and drawer locks, and buy bicycle helmets and crash-proof safety seats, but diseases and accidents still happen. Our children are exposed to the sadness and sorrow of bereavement when we would do all in our power to make them happy. In any discussion of grief, the bereaved or dying child is the most difficult to manage.

In earlier times, children lived with extended families and were aware of the death of family members at an early age. Many lived on farms and witnessed the deaths of livestock as a part of life. Today, death is usually removed to hospitals or is part of a television story that is no more real than the coyote who falls to his death, only to rise again in the next cartoon frame. Most children cannot understand that this is a cartoon and not real life. To protect children from grief, many well-meaning parents hide the death of a well-loved pet or quickly provide a replacement before the child has a chance to actively grieve for the one that died. They tell children that Grandmother is "sleeping" or "passed away," when the idea of passing away means nothing to the child. Trying to protect our children from the reality of loss may have kept them from developing effective coping mechanisms to withstand the shock of loss when it inevitably occurs.

With limited comprehension of the finality and the need for death, young children are less able to work through the task of grieving. If the loss involves a close family member, or

 LEGAL EAGLE

Patients have a legal right to limit medical intervention. Patients can complete an advance directive form that specifically says what actions are permitted and which ones cannot be performed. As a health care worker, you are legally obligated to follow the patient's directive. You may not agree with the patient's decision or wishes, but failure to follow the directive can result in fines and legal action against you and the health care setting. You must stay abreast of new laws pertaining to completing and documenting advance directive forms.

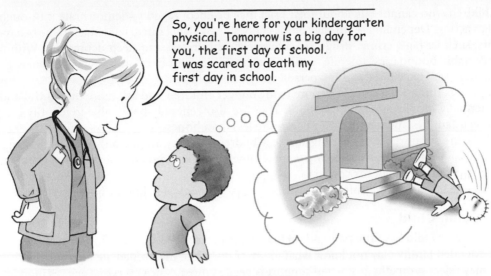

Figure 6-2

if a child is dying, the primary caregiver is also coping with bereavement and may have little emotional strength left to share. You may be the most available resource to help the child either work through grief or prepare for death.

How can we help children cope with grief? The following suggestions will help with both the dying and the bereaved child.

- Be honest. Speak of dying and death. **Euphemisms** such as "He is (or you are) going to a better place" or "She left us," etc, are confusing and leave the child wondering either why he cannot go also, or why he must go if he is the one dying. "This place" is the only place the child knows, the concept of a "better place" is frightening rather than reassuring. It may also imply that he or his loved one may be coming back. Even young children can be helped to understand that he or his beloved person will not be coming back but that this new place is free of pain and suffering (Fig. 6-2).
- Maintain routines as nearly normal as possible. Children need structure; it gives them a feeling of security.
- Expect regression to more dependent stages. Children who are grieving complain of headaches, nightmares, and phantom illnesses and may exhibit bed-wetting or poor school performance.
- Reassure children that this is not in any way their fault; it was not because of anything they did or did not do. Children are very egocentric, all of life revolves around their concerns; if this person died, it therefore must be the child's fault. If the child is dying, he or she feels this is punishment for being bad. Do what you can to help them cope with this natural feeling of guilt.
- Explain that it is normal to feel sad, lonely, or angry and that you may feel all of these things, too. Tell children that you are available when they want to talk and that it is OK to cry. Cry with children if they need to mourn; it validates their feelings.

- Children who cannot talk about their grief may be encouraged to demonstrate it through play-acting. Depending on the age of the child, some will act out grief with extreme behaviors, such as rage, crime, drugs, or, conversely, withdrawal and deep depression. Within acceptable boundaries, tolerate "acting out" hostilities and irrational behavior. It may be the only way the child or young person can express himself.
- Teenagers think for themselves more than younger children and ask more thoughtful and potentially more disturbing questions. They are also generally better able to identify evasions if families and health care workers are less than honest.
- Children's support groups are invaluable. Children feel they are the only ones in their age group to feel this way. Introducing them to other children who are grieving gives them an age-appropriate outlet for concerns.
- If all else fails to relieve suffering, professional psychological help may be necessary.

The Dying Child

Since a dying child has little past and no future, the present is even more important. Friends and extended family may not know what to say or do, while the immediate family is in crisis and may reject sympathy just when support is needed most. Since everyone grieves individually, family members usually are at different stages at a time they need to be in harmony. Families do better when they know what to expect, such as how much pain the child will experience and whether it can be managed, how debilitating it will be, how long it may last. The child also needs age-specific explanations. Children usually reflect their parents' emotions; for example, if parents are frantic and emotional, children pick this up quickly and reflect these emotions. Your most effective and therapeutic measure is to support and comfort parents to cope with the situation as calmly and with as much preparation as possible. Calm acceptance helps soothe the child.

In addition to the general suggestions outlined above, add these measures for the dying child:

- Remember to comfort siblings and families of a dying child. Other children in the family may resent the time and attention denied them and feel guilty about these perfectly natural feelings. Every family member, no matter how strong, needs comfort. Many families do not survive the death of a child. With a very sick child, expect a very troubled family.
- Teenagers are better able to visualize the future they will lose, which leads to more anger and depression than younger children experience.

The Bereaved Child

Children fear separation long before they know to fear death, and death is the ultimate separation. As with adults, how well children cope with bereavement depends on how much support they can expect from caregivers. Much of their adjustment is affected by the child's life experiences with other forms of losses, how many other stressors they have at this time, and so forth. If their home life is stable, supportive, and nurturing, most survive the experience without lasting trauma.

Helping children cope with the loss of someone or something significant in their life, even a loved pet, is challenging no matter what the child's age. It is somewhat easier with older children and teenagers than for young children with limited experience and comprehension; however, the following suggestions may help.

- Allow the child to grieve; it seems to reduce the fear of death for all age groups to work through the stages of grief.

- Discuss the cause of death in an age-appropriate manner. Use terms and examples children can understand. Be cautious of euphemisms; they can be very confusing.
- Allow but do not force children to attend funerals. When children resist, they are not ready; however, if they express curiosity and a desire to be part of the funeral, they may need the comfort of leave-taking rituals that help all of us through the process.
- Encourage questions, but do not press; simply be available when the child feels the need to talk.
- Talk about the person who died. It is healthy to remember good times and reaffirms love and affection. Encourage children to remember special times; if they are mature enough, it helps to write about memories and feelings to keep the love alive.
- If parents are dead or dying, encourage family members to discuss plans for the child's care as quickly as possible. Fear of "what will become of me" is very real to children. They need reassurance that they will be cared for and loved.

The recognition of death and the grief process must be reexamined with each new level of maturity and understanding. The boy who seemed to work through his grief at six may feel it again at puberty when his father is not there to guide him or to accompany him to sports events. A young girl may have to work through grief again at menarche without her mother and with no close female relative to discuss this transition with her. Preteen children may continue to wonder about death, with questions such as, "Does it hurt?" "Are animals there?" Many children and young people think death is a reversible process. The death of one teenager in a school or a group may lead to "cluster deaths" as others tempt fate by unwise choices. This dangerous trend must be guarded against with grief counseling. At each new age of awareness, children need to reconsider loss until they have matured through the process to acceptance.

Helping Adults Cope with Loss

Adults have more time to plan and anticipate their mortality as they experience the loss of health or death of their contemporaries. Adults usually have experienced many losses and have worked at coping with them realistically. Middle-aged and older adults either have accomplished most of their life plans or realized that they probably will not write the great American novel or be drafted by a major sports team. Many older adults have fewer pressing obligations, such as young children or career objectives, while young adults still have many responsibilities. Adults with good support networks and manageable stress levels grow through grief in time, although much depends on available family and friends for support. All of these considerations make discussing grief and loss with adults different than discussing it with children who have limited understanding.

Younger adults usually die of accidents or acute diseases with little or no time to plan. They may leave young children and complicated family affairs, which magnifies the grief response and makes survivor grief more intense. Older adults usually die of long-term degenerative diseases that allow years of preparation for loss. Older adults must also cope with many social losses and greater health challenges at a time when they have fewer support resources. They may have fewer available friends and distant families that are more involved with a growing family and career than with the aging parent. Older adults frequently have fewer financial and emotional resources but usually have less fear of death. Although communicating about death is easier with most adults than with children, where adults are in their life span has an impact on readiness to accept mortality.

Many of the points listed above for children are appropriate for all age groups experiencing difficulty in working through loss. The following suggestions also work for most situations:

- Find out what the patient and family know about the anticipated or actual loss. Never presume to educate either patients or family beyond your scope of practice, but help them plan for pain, debilitation, loss of mobility, and so on, as you are able.
- Establish trust and a good rapport early, so that patients and family feel comfortable talking with you and turning to you for assistance.
- Listen actively. Look for cues that you need to listen even more closely to what is not being said.
- Look for practical ways to help in addition to medical measures. In an inpatient situation, help patients and families gather laundry, tend gift flowers, and plan for home care; in an outpatient situation, you may help arrange transportation or make care simpler for home treatment.
- Validate the sufferer's feelings. Each participant has a right to his or her own fears and feelings. Concentrating on the loss may appear morbid, but for some people, it seems to help make sense of the situation and raise awareness of the loss so that healing can begin.
- Support the family's established faith and refer them to their spiritual leader.
- Help the family and patient gather together all available support, such as hospice and grief counselors.
- Allow as much control as possible. Let patients and family members make as many decisions as they feel comfortable making. During some levels of grief, the griever may have trouble making any decisions and will turn to you for help.
- Be there for them or give them as much privacy as they need. Be alert for cues for either need. You do not always have to *do* something to be helpful. Simply sitting in silence can be very calming.
- Encourage patients and family to express their grief but do not press the issue. Some people prefer to grieve privately and will be distressed if you pressure them to conform to your expectations.
- Help patients and family talk about the future and help them make realistic plans, but encourage them to talk about their memories; it helps them make sense of the loss. It is not unreasonable to ask a dying patient or the family members to recall youthful stories of careers, travels, homemaking, or "how-we-met." Memories can be very comforting.
- Encourage respite without guilt. Caregivers need time to themselves, and patients may also need time without hovering caregivers. A relief from closeness helps avoid burnout and reduces anger and depression.
- Talk with the physician if the patient or caregiver feels that needs are not met, such as pain relief or anticipatory education. Take advantage of every resource for assistance.
- When appropriate, show that you care by a touch, a hug, or a pat on the shoulder.
- Simply say, "I am so sorry for your loss." Do not try to be profound or philosophical. Statements such as, "He would not want you to grieve," or "She is in a better place," are not helpful.

Great loss does not happen in a vacuum; many persons are affected by the loss of one. Show you care by mentioning the deceased and remembering good things. You may say, "Mr. Jones, I am so sorry about Mrs. Jones. We always enjoyed visiting with her. I know you must miss her terribly." This will not renew Mr. Jones's grief—it never went away—but will reaffirm that other people miss Mrs. Jones also. A simple "I'm sorry" can let survivors know that you care and that they are not alone in their grief. Never say, "I know just how you feel," because you do not; each grief is intensely personal. And even though it may be so, never tell the survivor, "It was for the best." He may come to realize this, but it is not your place to point it out.

Protecting Yourself during the Grief Process

In health care, we tend to protect ourselves from grief by detaching and viewing patients as disease processes when the pain of caring is overwhelming. Patients become "case studies." This detachment helps us avoid thinking about death. To avoid this detachment, we must face our own doubts and fears to help patients cope with their concerns. You must resolve your feelings about death and loss, or you cannot give effective care. Loss will hurt more if you care deeply about your patients; however, caring deeply *about* patients should not interfere with caring *for* patients. And remember that you have to go back tomorrow and do it all over again.

At times, the unrelenting pain of certain patients is overwhelming. This can be either the patient's emotional pain or physical pain that does not seem to respond to anything we do to help. For some, grief is so devastating that the process is intensified beyond our ability to offer comfort; some physical pain is so unbearable that our strongest narcotics are ineffective. We may dread contact with the grieving or suffering patient or family because there is nothing substantial we can do to help. In these instances, when our professionalism and all we have to offer is not enough, we may doubt ourselves and pull away from the sufferer. We look for reassurance in other situations that make us more comfortable; we turn to other patients who we know we can help. In these instances, you should step back emotionally, take a deep breath, and then move back closer in empathy to be available for whatever compassion you can offer. Under no circumstances should you abandon a patient or caregiver who seems beyond your ability to help, no matter how slight that aid may be.

The term "burnout" implies that your fire to help has gone out. This loss of enthusiasm for your profession is a high price to pay for caring. What can you do to make it easier to go back every day and practice your passion?

- Develop outside interests that direct your mind away from health care.
- Remember to protect yourself by taking time for yourself. Do things you enjoy away from the professional setting and do not feel guilty about it.
- Take care of yourself: rest, relax, and eat right.
- Read available literature regarding grief and "letting go." You will find helpful suggestions for yourself and your patients.
- Talk to your spiritual advisor about your doubts and fears. Determine why you are so affected or frightened by the prospect of this unavoidable life stage.
- Take comfort from your faith and your support groups of family and friends.

As we do everything in our power to help our patients, we must remember to care for ourselves. If we leave the profession because we can no longer give what it requires, not only will we lose, so will our patients.

WORKING WITH SUPPORT AGENCIES

Most communities have valuable, active groups to support patients and families who are experiencing grief and loss. If the loss involves health, but the patient is not terminally ill, most diseases and disorders have support groups to make adjustment less traumatic. These are called "befriender programs," and they call on others who have successfully coped with the changes to help make the transition to living with an illness. Types and levels of support groups are covered more fully in Chapter 4, "Educating Patients."

Support does not necessarily need to be an organized group; as noted in Chapter 4, a strong group of close friends can be just as effective. This is seen in groups of widows or widowers who meet and share grief and joy in their mutual circumstances. Many times, these groups are more supportive than formal groups of strangers, even with the common interest of illness. The familiarity of shared history with friends is very comforting.

If you are in the position of suggesting support agencies to patients and caregivers, remember that, as in all areas of medicine, not everyone has the same needs. Whereas some patients and families need and welcome the open sharing of support, others prefer to cope privately and are uncomfortable sharing deep personal feelings with groups, no matter how supportive the group may be. Patients and caregivers may attend a few times and decide they prefer to concentrate their energy in other coping measures. Some may complain that support groups focus on loss when these patients and family members prefer to focus on living. This may be particularly evident during the denial or anger stages. If most of the participants in the support groups are in depression or acceptance stages, those in other stages are less likely to find benefits in the group experience. As with all other coping measures, patients must make decisions that bring them comfort. Trying to force patients to participate in what we think is right will only increase stress.

For those who are expected to die within a certain time, the Hospice organization works with all family members to adjust to the approaching loss. Certain locations have hospice centers that are less medically oriented than hospitals but have workers trained to care specifically for the terminally ill. In areas without formal Hospice centers, the Hospice organization encourages the terminally ill to remain at home with only the technology the family or patient chooses. Specially trained volunteer workers discuss dying, death, funeral arrangements, financial concerns, and so forth. The Hospice organization oversees the training of its volunteers, coordinates and supervises patient and volunteer interaction, and helps provide equipment and supplies for end-of-life care (see Spotlight on Success box). Hospice offers **palliative** care, with an emphasis on comfort rather than cure. Palliative care respects the patient's choices in medical, emotional, social, and spiritual needs and supports the needs of the family. This form of care looks at the patient holistically, ensuring comfort and compassion with no medical measures against the patient's wishes. After death, Hospice volunteers are available to help survivors settle insurance, hospital bills, funeral matters, and legal issues. At a time when many friends of the family have said their goodbyes and returned to their normal life, Hospice is still available to help survivors with the task of healing. Your responsibility during this time is to support both patient and family with your medical knowledge and skills and, just as important, your care and compassion.

We have become members of the health care profession to help relieve suffering in all of its forms. When all that we know how to do is still not enough, and death is inevitable, our professionalism is put to its strongest test. It is in managing grief and loss that we prove to our patients and ourselves that we have made the right choice.

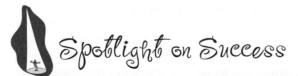

Spotlight on Success

Would you like credible medical experience to include on your resume? Think about becoming a Hospice volunteer. Volunteering is a great way to obtain experience and to network with working professionals. The roles and responsibilities of Hospice volunteers differ based on experience levels and background. You will be given a full orientation before starting and will be monitored throughout the process.

Taking the Chapter to Work

Now, let's meet Susan and see how she has applied this chapter information in the workplace. Susan is working in an obstetrical office. She is caring for a 42-year-old woman who was seen two nights ago in the hospital's emergency department for vaginal bleeding and cramping. The patient is 12 weeks' pregnant and has had three spontaneous miscarriages in the past. Susan recognizes that although the patient has not miscarried this pregnancy as of yet, the patient is at risk for perceived and anticipatory grief. Susan uses her communication skills to evaluate the patient's physical and emotional status. A few minutes later, the physician examines the patient and finds that the cervix is open and that a miscarriage is inevitable. The patient shouts out "No, this can't be. You are wrong." Susan recognizes this as a normal stage (denial) of grief and loss. Susan knows that support groups are available for women who have experienced miscarriages, but it would not be appropriate to give this patient these pamphlets at this time. Susan remains with the patient and offers support. She also offers to call the patient's spouse. Six months later, the patient returns to the office for a routine visit and thanks Susan for her caring and compassionate support.

Beyond the Classroom Exercises

Your Assignment Board

The following exercises will help you apply what you learned in the chapter. Place a check beside the assignments your instructor has given you. When you have completed the assignment, place a check in the completed column.

		Assigned	*Completed*
Checking Your Comprehension	(Textbook)	☐	☐
Expanding Critical Thinking	(Textbook)	☐	☐
Communication Surfer Exercises	(Textbook and Internet)	☐	☐
Communication Tree Branch #9	(CD-ROM)	☐	☐
Communication Tree Branch #10	(CD-ROM)	☐	☐
Patient/Caregiver Interview #5	(CD-ROM)	☐	☐

Checking Your Comprehension

Write a brief answer for each of the following assignments.
1. Define the term *thanatology*.
2. List and explain Engel's stages of grief.
3. List and explain Kübler-Ross's stages of grief.
4. Explain the difference between an actual and a perceived loss. Give an example of each.
5. What is a palliative treatment plan?
6. Define the term *euphemism*. Give five examples of euphemisms pertaining to death.
7. What does the term *burnout* mean? List five actions you can take to prevent it from happening to you.

Expanding Critical Thinking

1. If you found studying this chapter disturbing, describe your feelings as you worked through the subject.
2. In 50 words or fewer, explain how you feel about death. Consider death for yourself or for those close to you. Do you see death as a natural part of life, or do you avoid considering the prospect?
3. Do you fear the unknown, or do you have faith that only good will come to you after death?
4. If you knew the day of your death, would you live differently? If so, what would you do?
5. What do you want to accomplish before you die?
6. If you knew that you were to die soon, would you try to mend broken relationships?
7. How would you say "goodbye" to those you love?
8. How would you want those you love to say "goodbye" to you?
9. What technological measures would you refuse at the end (i.e., endotracheal tube, IVs, AED, chemotherapy), or would you request that every measure be used to keep you alive? Would you make the same choices for those you love?
10. How do you think your view of death differs from your parents, grandparents, or younger siblings?
11. Write your own obituary and epitaph.
12. Obtain a copy of your state's Living Will and Advanced Medical Directive. Read these forms and record your feelings.
13. How does your family grieve? How does this differ from your friends or classmates?
14. Compile a list of euphemisms for death that are common in your area, such as "He went to his reward," or " She was called home." Explain how these terms might confuse a child or someone who speaks English as a second language.

Communication Surfer Exercises

1. Make a list of common religious affiliations in your community. Select four different religions that you are not familiar with, then using the Internet, search for information about their beliefs regarding dying. How would your ability to communicate differ with each group? What barriers to communication could arise? How would you resolve them?

2. Select five cultural/ethnic groups and search the Internet for information about their burial beliefs. Assume a patient has died and the physician has ordered an autopsy to be done, but the family states that according to their beliefs the body needs to be buried within a certain time frame. How would you communicate the importance of an autopsy to the family? Write at least six statements or phrases that could help the situation and six statements that would make the situation worse. Compare your statements with your classmates.

3. Using the Internet, search for five sites that help parents cope with the loss of a child. Create a list of 10 communication tips from these sites. Now, search the Internet for sites that would help a child deal with the death of a parent. Create a list of 10 communication tips from these sites.

4. Find the Internet address for Hospice. What does Hospice do? What are the benefits to Hospice care? How would you communicate these benefits to a patient? What phrases could help? Where is the nearest Hospice center to you?

5. Locate five Internet sites that download advance directive forms. Print them. Now, bring them to class and role-play with a classmate. Explain what the form means and how to fill it out. How did you feel discussing this issue? Are you comfortable communicating about death and end-of-life care issues? If not, what steps can you take to increase your comfort level?

7

WRITTEN COMMUNICATION: IT'S MORE THAN JUST WORDS

LEARNING OBJECTIVES

Upon successfully completing this chapter, you will be able to:

- Explain the importance of written communication.
- Describe 13 guidelines for charting in a medical record.
- Describe the two common methods of organizing the medical record.
- Describe and give examples of narrative charting using the SOAP, SOAPIE, SOAPIER, and PIE formats.
- Explain how flow sheets, graphic sheets, and progress notes promote communication in a health care setting.
- Describe the practical tips for communicating specific issues on a medical record.

KEY TERMS

Abbreviation	Graphic sheet	Progress note
Consent form	Incident report	Reimbursement
Flow sheet	Noncompliance	Triage

Test Your Communication IQ

Before reading this chapter, complete this short self-assessment test. Decide if each statement is true or false.

1. Good charting skills are essential for legal protection and reimbursement of medical expenses.
2. It is not necessary to chart every normal finding, only abnormal ones, in a medical record.
3. Use abbreviations frequently in the medical record to save writing time.
4. The medical record is an important communication tool among medical professionals.
5. It is best to use many adjectives and to write lengthy descriptions about your patient. A longer note is more thorough.
6. It is okay to ask a friend to chart for you.

Results

Statements one and four are true. All others are false. How did you do? Read the chapter to find more information on these topics.

IMPORTANCE OF WRITTEN COMMUNICATION

While the physical and emotional care provided to patients is very important, the documentation of this care is essential. Documentation in the medical record is an important form of written communication. It serves many purposes. Listed below are some reasons that documentation is important:

- Continuity of care
- Legal protection
- Reimbursement
- Quality improvement
- Regulatory standards

Here is a closer look at each of these reasons.

Continuity of Care

The medical record is a communication device by which health care professionals share their knowledge, assessment, and care of a patient. It allows for continuity of care in the outpatient setting as well as in an inpatient setting. For example, in an office setting, the patient may be seen in January for an ear infection and not return to the office until late November for another ear infection. By looking back on the documentation of the January visit, the physician might select the same antibiotic that worked previously. Or, for example, the patient may have a serious wound infection that is not healing. By looking at the medical record and reading the documentation, a new team member can eliminate things that previously failed to work and then can recommend a different treatment.

Legal Protection

The primary evidence used in court is the medical record. In a trial, your written communication will either help your care or hurt it. The golden rule in charting is "If it was not charted, it was not done." Jurors from medical malpractice cases have been polled after the verdict has been rendered and the most important piece of evidence in their decision was the medical record.

You cannot depend on your memory to recall the facts. Malpractice suits often take years to come to trial. At minimum, you must document what was done, when it was done, who did it, and the patient's response to the treatment.

Reimbursement Documentation

Accurate written documentation communicates to insurance companies what care was provided and what supplies were used. Third party payers review the medical record to determine what supplies were used, if they were needed, or if the tests (e.g., x-ray, blood work) were necessary and delivered appropriately. After the review, the insurance company will decide if the medical setting is eligible for reimbursement. **Reimbursement** is the payment made by an insurance company to a health care setting for medical services.

For example, assume that a patient develops a moderate nosebleed and needs a posterior nasal balloon. The chart note stated, "Pt had a nose bleed. Pressure applied. Dr. Jones into see pt." Nowhere in the medical record did anyone document that a posterior nasal balloon was inserted. The third party payer can refuse to pay (reimburse) for the balloon costs.

Patient education must also be documented for the insurance company to reimburse the health care setting for this service. For example, assume that you are working in a clinic and spend an hour educating a patient about a particular skill. In some situations, the physician's office can bill the insurance company for that teaching. However, if the medical record does not reflect that the education occurred and the length of time, the insurance company will not reimburse for the education.

In the hospital setting, peer review organizations (PRO) will examine charts to determine whether the patient's length of stay was appropriate. Unless documentation supports additional hospital stay, the institution or setting may not be compensated for the difference. For example, assume that Paula Morrello was admitted to the hospital for pneumonia. The morning that she was to be discharged, she developed a rash and thus was kept overnight for observation. According to the Diagnostic Related Groups (DRG) (Box 7-1) standards, patients with pneumonia should be discharged in 3 days, but because of this rash this patient remained in the hospital for another day. Unless the documentation clearly states the need for the additional hospital stay, Medicare will not cover the extra day in the hospital. It will claim that it was simply "an allergic rash and that the treatment could have been

Box **7-1**   **DRG Definition**

The Diagnostic Related Groups (DRG) is a system in which hospitals are paid for services based on a precalculated structure. Under this plan, hospitals are paid a set fee for treating a patient regardless of the actual cost. The costs are determined by the patient diagnosis, age, gender, and presence of complications. Each diagnosis is assigned a "standard" length of hospital stay and a "standard" dollar amount. If the hospital spends more money than the "standard," the hospital loses that difference. However, if the hospital spends less money than the "standard," then the hospital keeps that difference. DRGs affect only inhospital care of Medicare patients.

managed at home" and the hospital will lose that money. Make sure you document any change in the patient's condition that would warrant a change in the plan of care.

Quality Improvement Data Collection

Health care settings look at medical record documentation for quality improvement purposes. Quality improvement is the process of identifying a problem, educating staff about the problem, and then reevaluating to see if the problem has been improved or resolved. Quality improvement programs are required by many regulatory agencies. For example, assume that you are working in an outpatient clinic and your supervisor has reviewed medical records and identified that "allergies to medications are not being documented." She can create a quality improvement program to fix this problem. She would start by communicating this problem to her staff and explaining why charting this information is important. And then, she would review new charts to see if the problem has been corrected. If the problem has not been corrected, she could do additional staff education or impose disciplinary action.

Staffing and budgetary needs can also be evaluated based on documentation. For example, assume that you are working in an outpatient mental health clinic that has two shifts (days and evenings). By comparing the number of patient visits and procedures done on various shifts, the supervisor can request more staffing during peak hours.

Regulatory Requirements

Regulatory agencies review medical records for documentation accuracy. They review medical records because documentation is an essential component of communication in the medical community. Failure to properly document in the medical record can result in fines and loss of certification to a health care setting. The types of regulatory agencies that affect your job will vary based on your job title and employment site.

ESSENTIAL GUIDELINES FOR CHARTING IN A MEDICAL RECORD

There are many rules you must follow when writing in a medical record. Everyone must follow these guidelines to prevent communication mishaps. Here are the most common rules and some examples showing how communication mishaps can occur.

Use Military Time

Many health care facilities require that time entries be listed in military format. Military format is a 24-hour-clock system that allows each hour to be listed clearly without the confusion of a.m. versus p.m. (Fig. 7-1). Following is an example of a communication mishap that can occur when military time is not used. Which charting example gives a clear picture of when the patient fell?

Example # 1 – 1:20 patient was found on the floor.

or

Example # 2 – 1320 patient was found on the floor.

Example # 2 does not leave any doubt in the mind of the reader that the patient fell at 1:20 in the afternoon. The lack of documenting the abbreviation "p.m." led to the confusion.

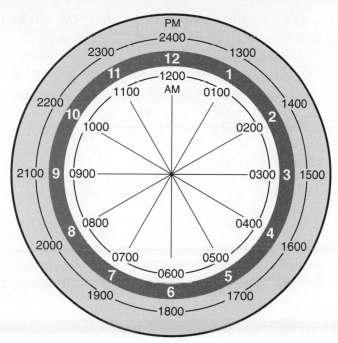

Figure 7-1
Military time. (From LaFleur Brooks, M., & Gillingham, E.A. (2004). *Health Unit Coordinating* (5th ed.). St. Louis: Saunders.)

Use Approved Abbreviations and Symbols

Abbreviations are short cuts to writing a complete word or phrase. When used correctly, they can save time, but if used incorrectly they lead to confusion. Incorrect abbreviations have led to errors in surgery (wrong limbs removed), wrong dosages of medications ordered or given, and incorrect tests or therapies initiated or cancelled.

On January 1, 2004, the Joint Commission on Accreditation of Healthcare Organizations (JCAHO) released new standards regarding the use of abbreviations within health care settings. These standards were developed to improve patient safety. Table 7-1 lists the abbreviations that may *not* be used. It is important to stress that this list changes periodically and the standards are updated frequently. It is your responsibility to remain current. Failure to comply with JCAHO standards can result in fines and loss of an institution's accreditation.

In addition to the above JCAHO standard, all health care settings, both inpatient and outpatient, are required to have a policy stating which abbreviations can be used and what the abbreviation means at that institution. Failure to follow the policy can affect your performance evaluation, your job security, and, most importantly, the patient's safety.

Symbols can also save time. Common symbols are > (greater than), < (less than), ♀ (female), and ♂ (male). These must be listed in the policy manual as well.

Table 7-1   JCAHO ABBREVIATIONS: ABBREVIATIONS THAT MAY NOT BE USED

Official "Do Not Use" List[1]		
Do Not Use	**Potential Problem**	**Use Instead**
U (unit)	Mistaken for "0" (zero), the number "4" (four) or "cc"	Write "unit"
IU (International Unit)	Mistaken for IV (intravenous) or the number 10 (ten)	Write "International Unit"
Q.D., QD, q.d., qd (daily)	Mistaken for each other	Write "daily"
Q.O.D., QOD, q.o.d, qod (every other day)	Period after the Q mistaken for "I" and the "O" mistaken for "I"	Write "every other day"
Trailing zero (X.0 mg)* Lack of leading zero (.X mg)	Decimal point is missed	Write X mg Write 0.X mg
MS	Can mean morphine sulfate or magnesium sulfate	Write "morphine sulfate" Write "magnesium sulfate"
MSO_4 and $MgSO_4$	Confused for one another	

[1]Applies to all orders and all medication-related documentation that is handwritten (including free-text computer entry) or on pre-printed forms.

*Exception: A "trailing zero" may be used only where required to demonstrate the level of precision of the value being reported, such as for laboratory results, imaging studies that report size of lesions, or catheter/tube sizes. It may not be used in medication orders or other medication-related documentation.

Additional Abbreviations, Acronyms and Symbols (For possible future inclusion in the Official "Do Not Use" List)		
Do Not Use	**Potential Problem**	**Use Instead**
> (greater than) < (less than)	Misinterpreted as the number "7" (seven) or the letter "L" Confused for one another	Write "greater than" Write "less than"
Abbreviations for drug names	Misinterpreted due to similar abbreviations for multiple drugs	Write drug names in full
Apothecary units	Unfamiliar to many practitioners Confused with metric units	Use metric units
@	Mistaken for the number "2" (two)	Write "at"
cc	Mistaken for U (units) when poorly written	Write "ml" or "milliliters"
μg	Mistaken for mg (milligrams) resulting in one thousand-fold overdose	Write "mcg" or "micrograms"

Following is an example of a communication mishap related to abbreviations. This sentence was charted; "Pt had normal bs this pm." What was normal this morning?
- blood sugar
- breath sounds
- bowel sounds

The answer is unclear and ambiguous.

Here is another example. What does the abbreviation pm mean?
- Per mouth
- Per month
- Per minute
- Post meridian

If you are using abbreviations, be sure to use only ones acceptable at your health care setting, and write them neatly.

Use Correct Punctuation

The placement of a comma or period can completely change the message. Pay special attention to punctuation marks. Following is an example of a communication mishap related to the lack of a period.

This sentence was charted; "Foley catheter removed in cardiac chair reading a magazine." Where was the Foley catheter removed ... in the cardiac chair? In reality, it should have been recorded: "Foley removed. In cardiac chair reading a magazine." It may seem a small mistake, but imagine defending yourself in court that you removed the catheter in bed and then put the patient into the chair. It is important not to leave any potential area for confusion or speculation.

The lack of a period or a period in the wrong place can lead to serious patient injury. For example, assume that you are working in an outpatient clinic and chart that you gave the patient 25 milligrams of a medication. However, the correct dosage was 2.5 milligrams. You may actually have given the correct dosage, but you charted it incorrectly. From a legal standpoint, you gave the patient 25 milligrams. The difference between those two dosages can be fatal.

Use the Active Voice

When writing in a medical record, use the active voice. An active voice conveys a natural and direct portrayal of events. The passive voice is an indirect and obscure recording. For example, "dressing changed" (passive) should be written as "changed dressing," which is in the active voice. Rather than writing "Dr. Rodriquez contacted," write "Contacted Dr. Rodriquez." An easy way to remember this is to start your charting sentences with a "verb."

Spell Correctly

Errors in spelling are unacceptable. They convey unprofessionalism, laziness, and poor judgment.

This sentence was charted: "A fowl smelling drainage was noted." Was the drainage foul smelling or did it smell like a fowl? The answer may seem obvious, but a prosecuting attorney will be able to place doubt in the mind of the jurors. Here are a few examples of spelling errors:
- Patient has *linguine* hernia.
- Mother states child not taking *foot* by mouth.
- *Fecal* heart tones heard.

Medications can have similar spellings but can have completely different actions. This sentence was charted: "pt was given Vepesid," but "Versed" was ordered. Vepesid is an antineoplastic medication and Versed is used for sedation. While you may have actually given the patient Versed as ordered, that was not communicated in the medical record. Remember: your written word is fact in the court room, with the insurance company, and in the eyes of your supervisor.

Be Concise

It is not necessary or recommended that you write lengthy narrative notes about normal events in patient care. For example, if an inpatient ate all of his lunch, you can simply write, "tolerated full lunch without problem." It would not be appropriate to write, "patient ate $^1/_2$ a bologna sandwich, three bites of an orange, 6 ounces of milk, and cup of unsweetened coffee," unless this was an unusual occurrence for the patient that required full documentation.

In a physician's office it would be appropriate to document that "Blood sugar log reviewed for March. Values ranged from 110-220." It is not necessary to record all the dates and their individual values.

Be Specific

Words such as *disoriented* and *confused* are vague and can be misinterpreted. For example, a patient can be "confused" when he calls you "Brenda" and not "Bonnie" but can still be well oriented to person, place, and time; he is simply forgetful, not confused. The treatment and cause for confusion is very different than the treatment for forgetfulness.

For example, the chart notes state: "patient was uncooperative." This phrase leaves many questions in the mind of the reader:
- What were the uncooperative actions—spitting, pushing, or fighting?
- Why was the patient uncooperative? Was he in pain? Were you giving him an injection? Was he confused?
- Did his actions affect patient care—did he refuse his pills, pull off his dressings, or refuse blood work?
- Was he uncooperative at every visit, or on every shift, or just this one time?

A better sentence to communicate what actually happened would be, "Patient stated that he didn't want to have any more finger sticks," and then record that the importance of blood sugar testing was explained to the patient and the physician was notified.

Be careful using "nonspecific" terms like *large* or *small*. For example, assume that you are working in a pediatrician's office and a mother arrives with her 6-year-old child. The child has a laceration on her leg. Which statement communicates the best information:
- Large laceration to left knee.
- Three inch laceration to left knee.

Use measurements when possible. Terms like *large* and *small* are very subjective. A mother may state that there was "large amount of blood," but in reality there was only a half a cup of blood. Ask patients for clarification when they use vague terms.

Write Legibly and Neatly

Poor handwriting is inexcusable and very unprofessional. The purpose of a medical record is to communicate information between health care providers. When an entry is not neat or legible it serves no purpose. For example, (T)s that are not crossed look like (l or L)s and

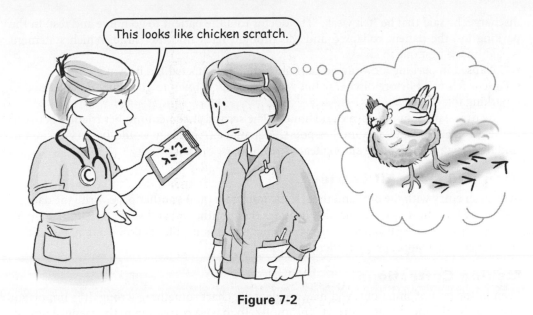

This looks like chicken scratch.

Figure 7-2

small (i)s that are not dotted look like (l or L)s. Small (e)s that are not made correctly can look like (c)s or poorly made (a)s can look like (o)s.

This sentence was charted: "line test done" but should have said "tine test done." An insurance company that audits this chart will not pay for this procedure.

Your signature must also be neat and legible. A sloppy signature does not portray professionalism (Fig. 7-2).

Organize Your Information

Always chart in a chronological order. Events that are not charted in this order lead to confusion and misinterpretation. These sentences were charted: "Dr. Brown notified stat. Ambulance called. IV started. Patient had seizure in waiting room." From reading this entry, it would have to be assumed that the patient had a seizure after the ambulance and after the IV was started. Questions could arise about the start of the IV and if any medications were given into the IV that caused the seizure. But in reality, this is what happened: "Patient had a seizure in waiting room. Dr. Brown was notified. IV started. Receptionist called the ambulance." This entry gives a clearer picture of the sequence of events.

Stick to the Facts

Do not put your personal assumptions or bias into charting. Just state the facts.

This sentence was charted: "Patient had not bathed in weeks, which caused the leg ulcer to get worse." This sentence is unprofessional and draws a conclusion about the patient's bathing regimen and hygiene. Unless the patient stated that he had not taken a bath in weeks, you cannot make that assumption. A better documentation would be, "Stage 3 lower left leg ulcer noted. Patient states that has not bathed because the shelter has closed."

It is never appropriate to use the medical record to criticize other professionals or to imply staff incompetence. For example, assume that you are working in an outpatient surgical clinic and you are caring for a patient that came in for a hemorrhoidectomy. Just before discharge, he said that he "felt weak." The doctor told the patient to go home and rest. In the parking lot, the patient collapsed and was brought back into the clinic. Which statement would be the best one to chart:

- Collapsed in parking lot. Brought back into clinic. Contacted Dr. Brown."
- Patient felt weak before discharge but was told by Dr. Brown to go home. He collapsed in parking lot.

The first statement is accurate and honest. The second statement implies friction between the team members and also implies poor judgment. An attorney would be very excited to find discrepancy or fighting among team members.

Sign and Date All Entries

Start each entry with the date and time. If the note goes onto another page, write the date on the top of that sheet as well. The date includes the month, day, and year (10/03/05). Sign all entries using your legal name. Make sure your name is legible. Follow your name with a comma and then appropriate credential initials.

Making Corrections

Even in the best of situations, you may accidentally chart something wrong. It is important to recognize the mistake and correct it promptly. To make a correction to the medical record, follow your office's policy and procedure manual. This is the standard method for making corrections:

- Draw a single line through the error. The error should still be legible.
- Write "mistaken entry" above or near the cross out. The term *error* is discouraged because it implies an error in care was made. You must follow your office policy.
- Make the correction as close as possible to the original entry. Be sure that it is neat and legible. Do not cram it into a small spot that cannot be read.

  Here are a few other important points to remember about making corrections:

- Never use correction tape or fluid.
- Never completely black out the mistaken entry.

  Box 7-2 has additional tips on documentation.

Making Late Entries

Late entries occur for various reasons. The two most common reasons are

1. The medical record is not available for charting. This primarily occurs within the hospital setting when the patient leaves the floor for tests.
2. The provider (you) forgot to chart something.

   To make a late entry, you must follow your office policy and procedure manual. Go to the appropriate area of the chart and enter the missing information. Write the present date and

Box **7-2** The Five Nevers of Documenting

Never document for someone else.
Never ask someone else to document for you.
Never document false information.
Never delete, erase, scribble over, or white out.
Never tamper with the medical record.

LEGAL EAGLE

Tampering with a medical record is illegal. Never assist or participate in rewriting documentation. There are many ways in which attorneys and law officers can detect a tampered medical record. Some clues of tampering are changes in the slant, pressure, or uniformity of handwriting; misaligned notations; and impressions or lack of impressions from writing instruments. Forensic experts can also lift up samples of the ink and test it to see if the same pen was used throughout the note. Experts can also use ultraviolet lights, infrared examinations, and other chemical tests to determine tampering. You can be fined, lose your license, and be terminated for tampering.

time. Then, write "late entry" with a brief note stating why this information was not charted. Start your note stating the time and date that the care was given. Record the appropriate information and sign the entry. Make your late entries as soon as possible. The longer after the fact, the more suspicious the late entry becomes (see Legal Eagle box). Here is an example of a late entry:

10/15/05 1300 Late entry: I forgot to chart this information. On 10/14/05 at 1500 elastic bandage applied to left foot. Toes warm to the touch. Able to move toes without problem. Ambulated to car using crutches. T. Williams CMA

ORGANIZATION OF THE MEDICAL RECORD

Generally, the medical record is organized into either of these systems: the source-oriented or the problem-oriented system. Here is a closer look at each system.

Source-Oriented Medical Record

This system was the initial organization of the medical record system. This system allows each medical specialty to chart its findings in its own section. For example, physicians chart their notes on the physician's progress notes, nurses chart on the nurse's note sections, and physical or respiratory therapists chart on physical therapy notes or respiratory notes, respectively. The chart is clearly divided by tabs.

Problem-Oriented Medical Record

Problem-oriented medical record (POMR), also called the problem-oriented record system (PORS), was designed in the mid-1900s and is one of the most popular systems used today. Most physician offices use this system. It divides the chart into four sections: database, problem list, care plans, and progress notes. All health care providers list problems on one problem list and then write a narrative note in the progress notes regarding the problem. This promotes interdisciplinary communication and teamwork.

COMMUNICATING THROUGH NARRATIVE NOTES

Two of the most common types of narrative notes are discussed here. The charting systems are discussed in their traditional format; however, there are multiple variations to these types and some health care settings have created their own versions. Your preceptor will explain the institution's policies. Below are the standard facts about these systems.

SOAP, SOAPIE, SOAPIER

Dr. Lawrence Weed wanted a uniform manner of documenting in the medical record. He created the SOAP format in late 1960s. It became popular very quickly and spread to nursing and other allied health care professionals. Over time, there have been numerous variations and adjustments. In its basic form, SOAP is written as follows:

Subjective (what the patient says): The patient's statement is written in quotation marks. The statement should be relevant to the topic of the note. For example, "My head really hurts" would be an appropriate quote if the focus of the patients visit was headaches, but it would not be an appropriate comment if the visit's focus was a leg ulcer.

Objective (what you observed): In this section, document your observations that pertain to the complaint. For example, "BP 180/134. Patient massaging temple regions of his head." A total head-to-toe assessment is generally not needed or appropriate. Only the abnormal or relevant (to the patient's complaint) are listed here. Vital signs are generally charted separately, except if they pertain to the complaint. Since a high blood pressure can be related to a headache, it is listed here.

Assessment (assessment or analysis): This is a phrase stating what you feel is wrong with the patient. It is not a medical diagnosis. For example, "leg injury" "laceration to right hand." You would not document "Strep throat" because that is a medical diagnosis, but you could write "Sore throat."

Plan (what you plan to do to correct this problem): For example, "Ice applied to left leg. Leg elevated on pillow."

Important: In some offices and health care settings, only the physician completes the assessment and plan section. The subjective and objective are completed by either nurses or other allied health care professionals.

SOAPIE and SOAPIER are two common variations of the above note. The "SOA" remains the same. The "P" focuses on what you plan to do, for example, "Will contact Dr. Constance." The rest of the record is written as follows:

Implementation (intervention or action that you performed): In this section, communicate to the reader the actual actions that you took for the patient. For example, "Tetanus 0.5 mg IM given in left arm."

Evaluation (patient response to the treatment): Here you document the patient's response to the interventions. In most cases, "SOAPI" is documented as one entry when the problem started, 0800, and then the E is added in as a later entry, 0930: "patient states my left leg feels better."

Revision (any changes needed or made to the implementation): If the evaluation did not show improvement, the R is added. For example, E: "leg pain is not improving." Then add R: "Motrin 600 mg given by mouth as ordered by Dr. Constance."

Remember: If you are working in any outpatient setting and give a patient a medication, be sure to document the patient's mode of transportation. Patients who are given any medications that alter their mental status or has possible side effects such as dizziness should not drive themselves home. Be sure to document the name of the driver.

PIE

The PIE charting format was created a few years after the SOAP format because some professionals felt that the SOAP format was too lengthy and needed to be more concise. The PIE format consists of only three letters and describes the problem, action taken, and then evaluation. Here is a closer look at PIE.

Problem (explanation of the problem): Unlike the S in SOAP, patient quotes are not always used, although some settings do allow and encourage them. The P is charted as "P: 'I fell last night.' Complaining of left leg pain. No swelling or discoloration noted. Small abrasion on left ankle."

Implementation (implementation or action taken): Left leg elevated on pillow. Abrasion cleaned with soap and water. Elastic bandage applied.

Evaluation (how the patient feels now and level of comprehension of teaching) Patient states "My leg feels better." Demonstrated use of crutch walking techniques without problem.

COMMUNICATING YOUR MESSAGE ON COMMON FORMS

Three common forms used for communicating between professionals are the progress notes, flow sheets, and graphic forms (see Spotlight on Success box). Following are some basic tips to remember when using these forms.

Progress Notes

Progress notes are lined pages that are used to document the patient's status and progress. The date and time are entered in the left column (Fig. 7-3). When using progress notes, you should do the following:

- Never leave empty lines. If there are only two or three lines on the bottom of the page, draw an X or lines through the empty lines and start on a new page. This prevents someone from tampering or adding additional information to the patient's record.
- If your note is going onto another page, on the top line of the new page, write the date and time, and indicate page #2. On the bottom of the first page write, "continued."

Flow Sheets

Flow sheets are used to document routine and repetitive actions. In an inpatient setting, they promote communication among different shifts. There are numerous types of flow sheets, but some common examples are flow sheets that document use of restraints, activities of daily living, range of motion exercises, safety assessments, and neurological checks. Depending on the type of flow sheet, the interval times can range from every few minutes up to 24 hours.

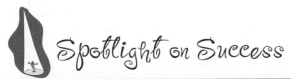
Spotlight on Success

Every health care setting has its own forms for documenting. Throughout your career, you will be exposed to many styles. It is your responsibility to read the policy and follow the instructions for using each style form. If a particular form does not seem to work well or is poorly designed, take the initiative and work on redesigning it. Ask your supervisor and team members for their input. Create a template and bring it to a staff meeting. Listen to their concerns and readjust the form. Enthusiasm and initiative are vital to future success.

PATIENT'S NAME_____   ☐ FEMALE   ☐ MALE   Date of Birth:_____/____/_____

DATE	PATIENT VISITS AND FINDINGS

ALLERGIC TO _____ PAGE_____of _____

Figure 7-3
Progress note form. (From Morton, T. (2004). *Kinn's The Medical Assistant* (9th ed.) St. Louis: Saunders. TM 66.)

In the ambulatory care setting, they promote continuity of care between visits. These flow sheets can be set up with intervals for days or months. Some common examples of flow sheets used in ambulatory care include medication, weight, and tracking the results of ordered tests.

Here are a few rules for using flow sheets:

- A change in the patient's condition requires a progress note to explain and detail the events.
- Make sure all boxes have an ✗ or ✔ (check) mark. If the box is not used or not applicable, a "N/A" should be noted.
- Most flow sheets require that you sign your full name only once at the bottom along with your initials. Only your initials are added next to the entries. If someone else has the same initials, be sure that it is clear whose initials belong to whom.

Graphic Sheets

Graphic sheets are used to document items such as vital signs or height and weight. It allows the reader to see the patient's progress at a glance. After the numbers are plotted on the graph, a line is drawn to connect them. The line should be drawn straight and solid. Use a ruler or other solid edge to make the line straight. If the patient's progress deteriorates, a narrative note should be written. It is important to communicate in the narrative note what actions were taken, when they were performed, whom you told about the changes, and the patient's response to the treatment.

COMMUNICATING SPECIFIC ISSUES THROUGH CHARTING

Depending on your job title and position, the specific care issues you encounter will vary. However, most specialties include these common tasks. Your supervisor or preceptor will give you more specific details, but listed below are some general guidelines to follow.

Admitting Patients

Most health care settings have specific admission forms to complete. Admitting forms are used in both inpatient and ambulatory care settings. Outpatient centers use these forms for patients who are coming in for 1-day surgeries. The purpose of the admitting form is to communicate to all health care providers the status of the patient's health at admission time. Some important information to communicate on admission includes the following:

- Chief complaint. This should be written in the patient's own words: "My stomach really hurts."
- Head-to-toe evaluation of all body systems.
- Complete set of vital signs.
- Medications taken at home; include the name of the medication, dose, and frequency. It is also helpful to communicate the level of understanding the patient has regarding these medications.
- Allergies to food and medications.
- Past medical or surgical history.
- Contact information.
- Insurance information.
- Any advance directives.

Discharging Patients

The discharge note must convey many things to the reader. First, the note must communicate that the patient is ready and safe to be discharged. When possible, a caregiver should be present to hear the instructions. Be sure to document the caregiver's full name and relationship to the patient. Other important aspects to communicate include the following:

- Any acute problems have stabilized and chronic problems can be managed.
- The extent and type of patient education.
- Patient verbalizes an understanding of the discharge instructions.
- Indication that the patient can self-manage or, if not, that help has been arranged.
- Medications, diet, therapies, wound care to be followed.
- Patient has safe place to go.
- Follow-up instructions. The date of the next appointment should be listed.

If the patient is being discharged from an inpatient care unit against medical advice, follow your medical center's policy manual. Most settings have a form the patient needs to sign that advises him of the risks of leaving against medical advice. Physicians must be notified of the patient's decision. Document all communication that took place between you, the physician, and the patient regarding this decision. Patients who are discharged against medical advice still must be offered education and resources for follow-up care. All attempts to offer these services must be documented, even if the patient refuses the services.

Physicians generally send a certified letter to any patient who leaves their office against medical advice. The physician may opt to send a patient-physician relationship termination letter.

Transferring Patients

Patients have the right to transfer to another physician or to another facility if they desire. Patients who decide to leave a physician for a new one should submit a letter communicating that they wish to terminate their relationship and that they want their medical records transferred to a given physician. Follow your policy and discuss this issue with the physician before copying and sending medical records to another physician.

Communicate these items in your discharge note for patients in a hospital setting who are transferring to another facility:

- Name of facility where the patient is going
- Mode of transport (private car, ambulance, helicopter)
- Evidence of communication with the receiving hospital that a bed is available
- A clear description of the patient's status
- Last set of vital signs
- Patient consent to be transferred

Call the receiving facility and verify the patient's arrival. Document that the patient arrived as scheduled.

Emergency Care

Depending on your specialty and place of employment, the type of emergencies that arise will differ. If you work for a family practice physician, you may encounter an elderly patient with a heart problem or a young child with a head injury that needs emergency care. If you work in an obstetrical office, you may have young women in premature labor. No matter what type of emergency occurs, always treat the patient first and then document the event. Communicate the following information in your narrative note:

- What happened
- When it happened
- What you did to treat the problem and any change in the patient's condition after your intervention
- Notification or presence of the physician
- Where the patient was sent after the event
- Notification of family members

Consent Forms

Patients must sign a **consent form** before any invasive procedure is performed. The consent form communicates to the reader that the patient has been told certain facts and agrees to have the procedure done. The legal implications of consents will be covered in your law and ethics course. At minimum, a consent form must include the following:

- Name of the procedure to be performed
- Date of the procedure
- Who is performing the procedure and any assistants
- Type of anesthesia to be used
- Statement that the risks and benefits of the procedure have been explained to the patient and the patient understands them.

A consent form is also required if a photograph is taken of the patient. Consent form signatures must have a witness signature. Follow your office policy regarding witnessing a signature.

Patient Education

Depending on your job and title, the amount of patient education that you will be involved with will vary. Chapter 4, "Educating Patients," discusses patient education in more detail. Although most patient education sessions are informal, it is very important to communicate in the medical record that the patient did receive patient education. The following points should be communicated in your narrative note:

- Who was present (e.g., patient and caregiver and the relationship to the patient)
- What was taught (e.g., medications, diet, exercise)
- How it was taught (e.g., demonstration, return demonstration, video, handouts)
- Length of teaching (e.g., 10 minutes, 30 minutes)
- Level of understanding (e.g., "Patient verbalized or demonstrated understanding")
- Plans for additional teaching/support groups (e.g., "Patient referred to diabetes support group." "Flyer with additional information given to patient.")
- If an interpreter was present, include his/her name and the language translated

Incident Reports

Incident reports communicate unusual events to supervisors, physicians, and risk management personnel. Communicate the facts in a truthful and detailed manner. Do not embellish or eliminate information. For example, if you gave the wrong medication, communicate the event. Do not hide the facts. State only the facts as you know them. For example: "patient found on the ground." Do not write "the patient slipped on the ice in the parking lot," unless you actually saw the patient slip on the ice. The patient could have fallen while running or could have been knocked down.

There are many reasons to complete an incident report. Here are some of the most common reasons to complete this form:

- Medication errors
- Patient, visitor, or employee falls
- Performing a procedure on a wrong patient or wrong area on a patient
- Incorrect surgical counts, sponges or instruments
- Employee needlesticks
- Unusual occurrences that need to be communicated to your supervisor.

Patient Noncompliance

The medical record must include factual information about patient **noncompliance**. Noncompliance is the failure to follow medical instructions that can lead to serious patient consequences. The information must be factual and not demeaning. For example, it would not be appropriate to say "patient is stupid and is not doing what he is told to do." Instead, you must document the facts. "Patient arrived for appointment with wound open." No dressing. States, "I didn't feel like putting the dressing on this morning."

Not returning for follow-up visits or the failure to keep appointments also indicates non-compliance and must be documented. If the patient fails to follow medical instructions and keep appointments and later sues the physician for malpractice, the charting of these events will be critical for the defense. If a patient cancels an appointment or fails to show, you should document the date and time of the appointment and a statement that he cancelled or did not show. Call the patient, and then document the call and the reason ("I forgot about the appointment"). Indicate whether another appointment was made or if the patient is refusing additional appointments. Alert the physician to these events.

Telephone Triage and Telephone Advice

Health care professionals who work in outpatient centers or physician offices are often involved in telephone triage. **Triage** is a process of determining the degree of sickness and placing the patient into an appropriate level of care. Telephone triage is very tricky because the health care professional must rely only on the information that the caller is giving. After determining the nature of the problem, you often need to give advice on handling the problem. In other courses, you will learn specific skills for triaging and giving advice, but be aware that this practice is highly risky and must be carefully documented. Document the following information:

- Date and time of the call
- Name of the caller
- Name and age of the patient (if different than the caller)
- Nature of the problem
- Severity of the problem
- Length of time the problem has been going on
- Any interventions that the caller has tried and the results of those interventions
- Any instructions that you gave the caller

- Follow-up plan for the problem along with the time frame. (Example: "If the vomiting does not stop within 24 hours, call the office for an appointment.")

This information is charted in the patient's medical record. If you are working at a clinic and the caller is not a patient, follow your office's policy. Some policies state that you cannot triage or give advice to nonpatients, but other facilities allow you to. If the clinic allows nonpatients to call, there should be a telephone triage log that documents the calls.

Taking the Chapter to Work

Now, lets meet Jennie and see how she has applied this chapter information in the workplace.

Jennie is working in an outpatient clinic. The physician saw Jennie at the desk and asked her to give Scott James an influenza vaccine and James Smith amoxicillin 250 mg by mouth. At the same moment, the receptionist asked Jennie to come into the waiting room to triage a patient with a nosebleed. The nosebleed patient needed immediate help and required about 15 minutes of care. Jennie felt rushed and went into the medication room and obtained a flu vaccine vial and the amoxicillin. Jennie asked a colleague which room "James" was in. She was told room 4. Jennie went into room 4 and gave the flu vaccine to a James Smith. And, then she went into room 3 and gave Scott James the amoxicillin. These medication errors were made because Jennie did not follow numerous office policies. Fortunately, neither patient suffered ill results from her mistake, but these errors never should have occurred. Jennie told the physician immediately and he examined both patients. Jennie documented the incident as follows: In James Smith's chart, the administration of vaccine was documented, and in Scott James chart, the administration of the amoxicillin was documented.

A few minutes later, the physician told Jennie that is was now safe to "readminister" the correct medications. She gave the correct medications to the correct patients. Jennie documented in James Smith's chart the amoxicillin and in Scott James's chart the flu vaccine administration. After the patients went home, Jennie completed an incident report. She recorded her actions, then the physician wrote his note.

The medical record must always communicate the facts in an honest and truthful manner. Neither Jennie nor the physician attempted to hide or conceal the error. They completed the incident report as per policy. The failure to complete or falsification of an incident report can result in disciplinary actions.

Beyond the Classroom Exercises

Your Assignment Board

The following exercises will help you use your new knowledge. Place a check beside the assignments your instructor has given you. When you have completed the assignment, place a check in the completed column.

		Assigned	*Completed*
Checking Your Comprehension	(Textbook)	❑	❑
Expanding Critical Thinking	(Textbook)	❑	❑
Communication Surfer Exercises	(Textbook and Internet)	❑	❑
Voice Mail Message #6	(CD-ROM)	❑	❑
Voice Mail Message #7	(CD-ROM)	❑	❑
Patient/Caregiver Interview #6	(CD-ROM)	❑	❑
Patient/Caregiver Interview #7	(CD-ROM)	❑	❑

Checking Your Comprehension

Write a brief answer for each of the following assignments.
1. List five reasons that charting is important.
2. Describe nine essential guidelines for charting in a medical record and give an example of a communication mishap when these guidelines are not followed.
3. How are medical records organized?
4. Define each letter in the SOAP/SOAPIE/SOAPIER/PIE charting formats.
5. What information is communicated through a graphic form?
6. List five things that must be documented regarding patient education.
7. What information is communicated through an incident report?
8. What is telephone triage? What items should you document after a telephone triage call?

Expanding Critical Thinking

1. With a partner, access surfer exercise #5 and then compare your forms. What are the strengths and weaknesses of the forms? Which form promotes better communication? Which form hinders communication? Now, create a new form.
2. Which medical record organization (source or problem) is better? Why?
3. Which narrative writing format promotes better communication? Why? Can you create your own acronym for charting?
4. Do you feel comfortable communicating with doctors through written communication? Do you think your spelling will affect your ability to communicate effectively? If so, how can you improve your spelling?

Communication Surfer Exercises

1. Go to the JCAHO Internet page. Find the standards for documenting in the medical record and print them. Find and print their standards regarding the use of abbreviations in a medical record.
2. Using the Internet, find your professional organization's home page. What standards do they have regarding charting?
3. Using the Internet, find 6 sites that can help you with spelling; two of the sites must contain common medical terminology.
4. Charting by exception and focus charting are two other less common charting formats. Using the Internet, find information about these two formats and write a brief description of each style.
5. Using the Internet, find a sample graphic or flow sheet used in a medical setting. Print the form and bring it to class to be used for a critical thinking exercise.

8

COMMUNICATING IN THE WORKPLACE: IT'S MORE THAN JUST PATIENTS

LEARNING OBJECTIVES

Upon successfully completing this chapter, you will be able to:

- Explain the concept of professional etiquette.
- Define the term *interdisciplinary communication*.
- Explain your role in participating in a case conference.
- Define the terms *emergent*, *urgent*, and *nonurgent* and provide an example of each.
- Describe common communication challenges and the strategies to overcome them when communicating with coworkers, physicians, managers, and regulatory agency personnel.
- Describe the guidelines for communicating with referral personnel.

KEY TERMS

Case conference	Emergent	Referral
Competency	Etiquette	Standard
Consultation	Interdisciplinary	STAT
Delegating	Nonurgent	Urgent

Test Your Communication IQ

Before reading this chapter, complete this short self-assessment test. Decide which statements are true and which are false.

1. It is permissible to call a physician "Doc"; this is friendlier.
2. You should never communicate with a regulatory agency investigator without the permission of your supervisor.
3. When discussing problems with coworkers, it is important to tell them how their behavior makes you feel and how it affects your ability to work.
4. Any sudden deterioration in a patient's condition is an example of an urgent situation to communicate to a physician.
5. As a manager, you should communicate sympathy and not empathy to your staff.
6. Phrases such as "that won't work" should be avoided when speaking to your manager.

Results

Statements three and six are true; all the other statements are false. How did you do? Read the chapter to find more information on these topics.

WORKPLACE COMMUNICATION: THE BASICS

The previous chapters have focused on communicating with patients. However, it is essential for you to develop a good rapport and communication pattern with your peers and other members of the health care team. Researchers have estimated that the average health care worker spends about 80% of his or her working hours communicating, and about 60% of that time is spent communicating with other health care professionals. Workplace communication must be professional and courteous and should be based on honesty and integrity.

Professional Etiquette

Etiquette is defined as the standard behavior that is acceptable in a given social, professional, or official setting. Standards of behavior are different for each of these settings. For example, if you meet a physician in a social setting, it would be appropriate to say, "Hi John," but in a workplace setting he should be addressed as Dr. Banks. Listed below are etiquette guidelines to remember in the workplace:

- Respect each person's knowledge and skill level.
- Accept each person's contribution to the health care team. No one person or specialty is more important than another.
- Workplace communication should be free from inappropriate topics, jokes, or betting. Ethnic/cultural jokes can easily be misinterpreted and therefore must always stay out of the work environment. Maintain patient and staff confidentiality. It is inappropriate to gossip or spread private information with other team members or patients. For example, it is unprofessional to say, "Did you hear that Dr. Raymond is getting a divorce?" or "I heard that he is involved in a big malpractice case."
- Always adhere to your professional organization's code of ethics.

Box 8-1   Health Care Specialties: Types of Health Care Professionals

Cardiopulmonary Technologist	Pathologist
Crisis Clinician	Pharmacist
Dietician	Phlebotomist
Emergency Medical Technician	Physician
Laboratory Technician or Technologist	Physician Assistant
Licensed Practical Nurse	Physical Therapist
Medical Assistant	Radiology Technologist
Medical Transcriptionist	Registered Nurse
Nurse Practitioner	Respiratory Therapist
Occupational Therapist	Social Worker
Paramedic	Speech Therapist/Pathologist

Interdisciplinary Communication

Communicating with various health care workers is termed **interdisciplinary** communication. Interdisciplinary is the combination of two or more specialties working together to meet a specific goal. The main goal of interdisciplinary communication is to promote optimal patient care. Each specialty (Box 8-1) provides a unique viewpoint and treatment plan for the patient and family. Interdisciplinary communication also

- Promotes teamwork, thus improving staff productivity and efficiency.
- Improves the patient care environment.
- Meets the requirements of various regulatory agencies.
- Helps to create or revise policies and procedures that affect more than one department.

    When communication is based on meeting the needs of a particular patient, it is termed a case conference.

Case Conferences

A common method for communicating about a particular patient is through **case conferences**. A case conference is a cohesive group of interdisciplinary professionals coming together to coordinate patient treatment. Case conferences start with each health care worker giving a brief summary of his or her clinical findings to the rest of the group. Discussion follows. Working together, the team prioritizes the patient's needs and creates a plan of care.

    A case conference can be formally organized or can be an impromptu meeting between professionals from different specialties. Formal case conferences are often planned and organized by the designated team leader. Generally, the team leader is the physician, case manager, or social worker. The team leader invites appropriate members of the health care team. Depending on the situation, a clergy representative, administrative staff, or regulatory personnel may be invited. In most cases, the patient or family is not present. However, depending on the case and the issues, the patient and/or family may be asked to attend a later portion of the conference.

    Case conferences can occur anywhere in the health care environment. They occur within hospital settings as well as in ambulatory care settings. The hospital's ethics committee may hold a case conference to discuss the removal of life support devices. In these situations, nonbiased, objective persons are designated to represent and speak on the patient's behalf. Legal council may also be invited to these conferences.

There are certain situations in which a case conference must be held. For example, in a long-term care facility, the Centers for Medicare and Medicaid Services (CMS) require an interdisciplinary case conference to be held periodically for any patient who is receiving Medicare benefits. There are specific guidelines for when and how often these conferences need to be held and who must attend. Medicare requires that a family member or significant other be invited to the meeting. Family members may decline to attend the meeting. Failure to hold these conferences and to document them properly can result in fines and potential loss of the right to bill for certain services.

During any case conference, communicate your clinical findings in an objective manner. It is never appropriate to gossip about the patient or family members or to let your own personal feelings or biases affect your clinical judgment. Any communication or discussion occurring in the meeting must stay in the room. It is not appropriate to discuss the meeting with anyone not associated with the case.

COMMUNICATING WITH MEMBERS OF THE HEALTH CARE TEAM

There are five specific groups of professionals with whom you must be able to communicate:
• Coworkers/peers
• Physicians
• Managers/supervisors
• Regulatory agency personnel
• Referral professionals

Each group is unique and comes with its own set of challenges. These challenges are discussed below, and some practical tips are also listed for each group.

Coworker/Peer

A coworker or peer is an individual with whom you work. Your job title may be the same, (Licensed Practical Nurse, Medical Assistant) but your roles and responsibilities may differ. This is related to factors such as level of expertise, experience, and seniority.

Communication Challenges

There are many potential challenges or barriers to communicating with coworkers. Listed below are some of the most common challenges:
• **Age:** Your coworkers may be younger or older than you. Differences in age may affect your ability to communicate openly and easily. Here are three examples showing how age can affect communication.
  • Newer medical terms replace older terms. For example, the term *nodal* (type of ECG rhythm) has been replaced by the term *junctional*; *rales* (type of breath sounds) are now commonly referred to as *crackles*.
  • Newer methods of performing standard skills can create challenges unless the health care provider attends continuing education courses. For example, "In CPR, we always gave five compressions to one breath for two-rescuer adult CPR. Who taught you

15 compressions to two breaths?" In this example, the provider took CPR in school years ago, but the ratios have changed.

- Age differences can limit our ability to feel like a member of the team. For example, if everyone you work with is younger or older than you, and they often socialize after work, your age difference may prevent participation. This may keep you from feeling like you are part of the team.
- **Different goals and objectives:** Everyone has different goals or objectives for working. Some of your peers may have hopes to become the next manager, whereas others may plan to retire in 6 months. Here is an example of how this can affect communication:
  - Jackie, who hopes to become the next assistant manager, is always thinking about ways to promote herself. She may start a conversation saying, "I think we need to redesign our documentation flow sheet."
  - Tonya has four children, works part time, and has no desire to expand her role. She quickly responds, "What is wrong with the one we have now?"
  - Jackie: "It's old and outdated"
  - Tonya: "Stop inventing projects. You are so difficult to work with."
  - While Jackie may have a valid point about the documentation sheet, these four sentences have left two coworkers at odds with each other.
- **Different work ethics:** Some people do 110%, while others opt to squeeze by at 75%. A statement such as, "When you see the gauze sponges are getting low, you should restock the wound dressing cart," can lead to a poor working relationship. Again, this may be a valid point, but it comes across as a negative statement and does not engage communication to resolve the problem.
- **Best friends:** A coworker can be your best friend outside of work, but in the work environment, you may come to resent covering your friend's inadequacies. Here is an example:
  - Sue: "I won't be able to get out on time and go shopping with you."
  - Barbara: "Why not?"
  - Sue: "Because I haven't even started charting yet and I have two medications to give."
  - Barbara: "How did you get so far behind?"
  - Sue: "I was trying to get a date with that new resident."
  - At this point, Barbara must decide whether to help her friend or go shopping alone. Helping out a best friend on a regular basis can strain any relationship and lead to the inability to work together effectively. This problem can be resolved easily with open communication about feelings and expectations.

Practical Tips

The remedy to all four of these challenges is clear and open communication. The failure to address or resolve any of these issues can have major effects on the work environment. Poor communication among coworkers leads to decreased productivity, poor patient care, and decreased morale. Below are some practical tips for promoting communication among your coworkers.

Use the acronym **PEER.**

Present the problem (explain the problem as you see it): "Today, *I* was trying to teach a patient how to use a home glucometer. We could hear your laughter in the hall."

Explain (explain how the problem makes *you* feel): "*I* felt really embarrassed when *I* was talking to the patient."

Effect (explain the effect the problem has on *your* ability to do *your* work): "It bothers *me* because *I* have to repeat my message and *I* feel that *I* have to apologize for the loud noise."

Resolve (explain that *you* want to resolve this problem so that *you* can work together better): "*I* really enjoy working with you and *I* want us to be able to work as a team, so *I* would like to resolve this problem. Can you try to lower your voice when sitting at the desk?"

Notice that throughout this communication the speaker emphasized "I." Starting a conversation by saying "You are loud," immediately sets the person referred to as "you" on the defensive. Focus on how it makes *you feel* and how *you* perceive the problem.

- Remember: there is a time and place for everything. Avoid any type of communication that may alienate a coworker or patient (Fig. 8-1).
- Humor can provide stress relief, but be cautious using it in the workplace. Appropriate humor may consist of a funny story or tale but must never include sexual or ethnic content. Practical jokes or setting bets is *not* appropriate in the workplace.
- Accept everyone. Value individual skills and strengths and accept weaknesses, and in turn, others will accept your strengths and weaknesses.
- Stay within your boundaries. It is not your job to discipline or reprimand another employee. The supervisor must handle these tasks.
- Never criticize or question a peer's performance or professionalism in front of other colleagues or patients. Instead say, "Before we leave today, I would like to talk with you about something. Can we meet in the lounge at 3 pm?" and bring the discussion into a private area.

Table 8-1 offers suggestions for phrases to use—and to avoid—when speaking with coworkers.

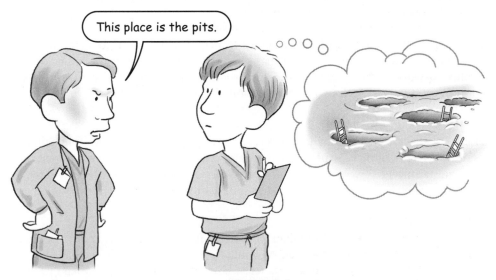

Figure 8-1

Table 8-1   Dos and Don'ts for Speaking with Coworkers

THESE PHRASES PROMOTE COMMUNICATION AND DIALOGUE.
DO USE THESE PHRASES:

"Lets talk about it."
"You did a great job with ...."
"Let's try it this way."
"I need some advice."
"How would you handle this problem."
"How can I help you?"
"I'll be free in 5 minutes to help you."

THESE PHRASES HINDER COMMUNICATION AND HALT DIALOGUE.
DON'T USE THESE PHRASES:

"Are you out of your mind?"
"You're lazy."
"You're crazy."
"You don't know what you are talking about."
"I can't help you."

Physicians

Guidelines for Contacting a Physician

All types of health care workers must communicate effectively and professionally with physicians or other patient care providers. Other providers include nurse practitioners, nurse anesthetists, and physician assistants. These professionals are ultimately responsible for patient care. For simplicity, we will refer to only the physician in this section, but keep in mind this includes any patient care provider.

Prioritize the nature of the problem. In certain situations, you should contact the physician **STAT** whereas in other cases, you may be able to e-mail or leave a voice message. STAT is a situation that requires immediate attention. To contact a physician STAT, the physician is usually paged or beeped. The nature and type of emergencies that you will experience depends on your job title, place of employment, job setting, and specialty. It is important for you to be able to determine the **emergent** situations in your particular job and the appropriate method of communication. Your clinical supervisor or preceptor will teach you specifics as related to your duties. However, there are some general guidelines that affect every health care worker.

Contact the physician STAT for situations such as the following:
- Life-threatening change in a patient's condition
- Sudden deterioration in a patient's condition
- Laboratory or radiology results that require immediate interventions
- Patient care concerns that require emergent care

Box **8-2**   **Definitions**

Emergent—A condition or situation that needs *immediate* attention. The failure to act quickly will probably result in a serious or untoward event.
Urgent—A condition or situation that needs *quick* and *prompt* attention. The failure to act within a reasonable timeframe could result in a deterioration of the patient's condition.
Nonurgent—A condition or situation that needs to be addressed but it is not time dependent. The outcome will not be worse if the condition is not resolved promptly.

Contact the physician (non-STAT) for situations such as the following:

• Clarification or changes to medications that are not life-threatening. For example, a patient may call the physician's office and tell you that his morning blood sugar was 210. The patient wants to know if he should increase his evening insulin dosage. This situation is not an emergency, but it must be handled in a timely fashion. If the patient had called the office reporting a very high or low blood sugar or was experiencing symptoms, then the physician would need to be contacted STAT.

• Patient care concerns that require **urgent** care. For example, a nurse from a skilled nursing facility has called a physicians office and told you that a patient has developed a new skin ulcer. This patient deterioration does not warrant an emergent page but needs to handled in a timely manner (Box 8-2).

Leave a message (e-mail, voice mail, or secretary) in situations such as the following:

• Normal laboratory or radiology results

• Positive patient care updates

• Patient or family/caregiver requests to speak with the physician about a **nonurgent** matter

Communication Challenges

There are many challenges or barriers to communicating with physicians. Following are some of the most common challenges:

• Intimidation—As a newcomer to the medical field, you may feel intimidated speaking with a physician. This is understandable and very common among new graduates. These feelings will subside as your experience level increases, your comfort level grows, and you become more acquainted with the physician.

• Different personalities—Each physician is an individual with a unique personality. Some physicians are very outgoing and happy to answer your questions, whereas other physicians may appear to be short tempered. Do not allow personality issues and reputation to interfere with the need to contact a physician. If you find yourself avoiding a physician, speak to your manager and create a resolution plan. You must work to overcome any communication obstacle.

Practical Tips

When communicating with a physician, use the acronym **DOCTOR.**

Describe (describe the problem): Use terms that you are comfortable using. For example, "Mrs. Brown came into the office for her weekly blood pressure check. She was complaining of feeling very weak."

Observation (explain what/when you observed this problem): "She arrived at 10 a.m. and was very unsteady on her feet."

Clinical signs/symptoms (explain the clinical signs that you are seeing): "Also, I noticed that she was slightly confused and very diaphoretic. She was pale. Her pulse was 84 and blood pressure was 100/60."

Treatment (explain any treatments you have started or performed): "Since she is a diabetic, I checked her blood sugar and found that it was 40. I gave her a glass of orange juice."

Observations (describe any changes since the treatments): "She is more alert now and her blood sugar is now 80."

Request (ask the physician for treatments or changes to the plan of care): "Her daughter drove her to the office. Do you want her to stay until you come back into the office or can she leave with her daughter?"

By following this acronym, you will provide the necessary information to the physician in an organized and professional manner. Before the physician can make changes to the patient's medical regimen, he or she needs a thorough understanding of what is happening to the patient, when the change occurred, and what treatments have worked or not worked. Upon hearing this information, the physician can then decide to order tests, change medications, or initiate other treatment options.

It is very poor and unprofessional communication to say to the physician, "Mrs. Brown does not look good. Something is wrong." Physicians who feel they must draw each piece of information from you will become irritated and frustrated. Frustration is a barrier to positive communication.

- Treat the physician with respect. Respect is a two-way process. If you respect the physician for his knowledge and skills, the physician in turn will respect you and your skills. Respect is a trait that grows with time.
- Plan your communication. Planning what you need to say saves time. Talk with the physician when you have all of your facts in a concise order. Do not page the physician when you know that you are going to be busy with a patient and not able to answer the call. After paging the physician, alert the secretary that you have paged a particular physician. This prevents this scenario: the physician calls the office, and the receptionist has to say, "Who paged Dr. Rogacne? He's on line 2." Minutes go by, you are busy attending to another patient problem, and the physician is waiting, getting upset, and a barrier has been created before the communication even starts.

Managers/Supervisors

Guidelines for Contacting Managers/Supervisors

You must be able to communicate openly and freely with your manager or supervisor. You should feel comfortable speaking about many different topics, such as policy and procedural issues, staffing problems, or workplace environment concerns.

There may be times that you will need to discuss personal information with your supervisor. Personal issues that may affect your ability to work at your best level should be discussed with your supervisor before your work is affected. Discuss scheduling changes as soon as possible.

The method of contacting your supervisor will depend on his or her availability and your work schedule. Supervisors who are not immediately available will have beepers, voice mail systems, and e-mail access. Determine the most appropriate method for contacting them based on the topic and its urgency. The following issues warrant an emergent page:

- Unannounced or unplanned regulatory agency inspection
- Patient care situations that are unusual or need immediate attention
- Life-threatening patient care issues related to adverse medical treatment or an unexpected patient reaction

These situations require an urgent page:

- Procedural questions or concerns that require a prompt answer
- Immediate or upcoming staffing problem
- Any time an incident report needs to be completed

These situations could be handled as needed, or with a voice mail or e-mail message:

- Scheduling concerns or requests for future leave time
- Quality improvement ideas or suggestions

Communication Challenges

- Off Shifts and Off Site—Although some medical settings have established business hours, with employees and employers on site at the same time, there are many medical facilities that operate 24 hours a day, 7 days a week. You may work nights, or just weekends, and have very limited access to your supervisor. Some supervisors are responsible for various site locations and you may work at a satellite office and rarely actually see her. It is difficult to develop a communication rapport with someone when time and access are limited.
- Age—Whether you are younger or older than your supervisor, age can affect your ability to communicate. When supervisors are older than you, you may perceive them as "out of touch with reality," or view them as "old school." Conversely, supervisors who are younger than you may be perceived as "lacking clinical experience" and you may find it difficult to respect them.
- Unpopular decisions—Occasionally supervisors needs to make unpopular decisions. Most of the unpopular decisions are due to budgetary constraints or other regulatory mandates.

Failure to overcome any of these barriers affects your ability to communicate successfully with your supervisor. All of these issues can be resolved by using these communication strategies.

Practical Tips

Use the same PEER acronym that you used when speaking to a coworker, with the following modifications.

Present the problem (Present *your* problem. You should not try to explain someone else's problem.): " *I* noticed *I* am scheduled to work the afternoon shift 5 days next month and it is always on a Tuesday." Avoid stating the problem in an accusatory manner, such as "Why does no one else have to work Tuesday afternoons." Keep the conversation focused on *your* needs.

Explain how it makes *you* feel: "*I* understand that afternoons need to be covered, but it is hard for *me* to work late on Tuesdays because *my* daycare closes early on those days." Do not use words or phrases such as "This is not fair." Keep the conversation on *you* and how it makes *you* feel.

Effects (explain the effect the problem has on you): "*I* feel very stressed when *I* work on Tuesday afternoons because *I* feel rushed and anxious about my mother babysitting for *my* three children."

Resolve (You must be able to offer a solution that will meet everyone's needs and not just yours): "My daycare is open late on Mondays, so I would like to offer to switch my Tuesdays for someone's Mondays. Can I create a sign-up sheet to change the schedule?" Do not demand that the problem be resolved or make a statement such as, "You need to fix this problem or else!"

Notice the conversation dialogue focuses on the word "*I*" not on someone or something else. You may feel the schedule is unfair and feel tempted to place blame, but by focusing on you, the manager will be able to address your needs.

- Be organized. When you speak to your manager, have a list of key points that you wish to discuss. Start the conversation by saying, " I would like to talk about three things. They are …" and then begin with the main issue. Do not sound vague or unclear; for example, do not say, " I think there is a problem with this schedule." If you think you need more than 15 minutes to discuss your concerns, schedule an appointment with your manager. Scheduling an appointment demonstrates courtesy and allows for the manager to give you her full attention.
- Use written or e-mail message options. These methods save time and are often more productive than one-on-one meetings.
- Never blame particular individuals for problems. State the facts. For example, "The last 3 days I worked, I had to do all the Quality Improvement sheets. It makes me feel frustrated." Then continue with PEER. Avoid accusing anyone, such as "Michele has not done QI sheets in over a week." Trust your manager to understand and take action.
- Before entering the manager's office, knock on the door and ask permission to enter. Be aware of your kinesics and nonverbal cues.

Table 8-2 offers suggestions for phrases to use and to avoid—when talking with your manager.

Table **8-2**   **DOS AND DON'TS FOR SPEAKING WITH MANAGERS/SUPERVISORS**

THESE PHRASES PROMOTE COMMUNICATION AND DIALOGUE. DO USE THESE PHRASES:

"You can count on me."
"You have a good point."
"Thank you for this opportunity."
"I have given some thought to our problem and this may work…"
"I have an idea on how we can better use our resources."

THESE PHRASES HINDER COMMUNICATION AND HALT DIALOGUE. DON'T USE THESE PHRASES:

"It's not my job."
"It's not my fault."
"I've had it."
"This is a waste of time."
"I'm only human."
"I know who did that."
"It won't work that way."

Regulatory Agencies

Common Regulatory Agencies

To ensure consistent, quality patient care, the health professionals and their institutions (clinics, offices, hospitals) are among the most highly regulated agencies. Regulations come from four different areas: federal, state, local, and private. Federal laws are written and enforced by the highest governmental offices. State and local laws are often based on the federal law. Each type of law is assigned to a particular agency. Agencies are responsible for hiring investigators to enforce their laws. See Table 8-3 for a list of common regulatory agencies.

Investigators make site visits and look for evidence of compliance. Certain agencies send investigators on a regular basis (annually, semiannually) whereas others send an investigator only after a complaint has been filed. Some agencies visit without prior notice and others send documentation stating the date and time of the visit. Failure to prove compliance

Table 8-3   Types of Regulatory Agencies

Centers for Disease Control and Prevention (CDC)	Federal—Located in Atlanta, GA, www.cdc.gov	Responsible for tracking all types of diseases and illnesses. Also promotes education programs and preventing diseases. Good resource for vaccine-related information.
Centers for Medicare and Medicaid Services (CMS)	Federal with state offices www.cms.hhs.gov	Regulates Medicare and Medicaid funding programs. It also monitors and controls HIPAA and CLIA regulations.
Department of Public Health (DPH)	State, local—To find your state's Department of Health, go to a search engine and type the name of your state and then "health department"	Responsible for tracking various diseases in the state, promoting and ensuring safety of health care institutions within the state, regulating licenses of health care providers.
U.S. Food and Drug Administration (FDA)	Federal (Rockville, MD) with regional offices www.fda.gov	Responsible for drug manufacturing, prescription control; regulates medical devices.
Joint Commission on Accreditation of Healthcare Organizations (JCAHO)	Private—Located in Oakbrook, IL www.jcaho.org	Sets and enforces standards for health care institutions. Issues accreditations to health care institutions.
Occupational Safety Health Administration (OSHA)	Federal—With state offices. Federal office located in Washington, DC www.osha.gov	Responsible for ensuring workplace safety for employees.

during a visit (unannounced or planned) can have serious repercussions for the health care setting. Fines can be assigned and facilities can lose their license to operate under that agency. It is your job to communicate to the investigator that your health care setting is in compliance.

Guidelines for Contacting Regulatory Agencies

After you are hired, take the initiative to learn what regulatory agencies affect you and your position. Ask your manager questions such as, "What agency or agencies supply us with a license to operate?" "When can we expect to be inspected?" "What regulations/laws should I be familiar with?" A good policy and procedure manual will answer most of those questions. If you are hired into a hospital setting, you will be required to attend a hospital-wide orientation process where most of this information will be explained in detail.

Most agencies have a list of "reportable incidents" and the time frames for making reports. For example, the Centers for Disease Control and Prevention (CDC) has a specific list of communicable diseases that must be reported. Your local health department also has a list of communicable diseases that need to be reported and their time frames.

Each state has a division responsible for receiving and investigating suspected and confirmed cases of child or elder abuse or neglect. There are time constraints on these reports as well. Generally, an oral report is required within 24 or 48 hours, followed by a written report within 5 to 7 days. Failure to report and fill out these forms within the specified time can result in fines to the health care agency and to you personally and, in certain cases, even a reprimand on your professional license.

Each agency has its own forms that need to be completed and has instructions on how to make a report. Most agencies have a 24-hour number available for questions. All agencies have contact information on their Internet site. Remember, it is your job to know the regulations that affect you and your position, and it is your responsibility to remain current on the changes.

Communication Challenges

You will face many challenges when communicating with a regulatory agency investigator or representative.
- Confusing standards/language—The first challenge is understanding the **standard** and the language within the standard. A standard is a specific regulation or statement that is written by an agency and depicts the minimum level of expected care. Standards are sequentially written and organized by a series of numbers and letters. For example, the investigator may say to you, "I need to see your action plan for compliance with standard 256B, subsection 67.39, Part III, version B." Unless you are very proficient with the standards, you may feel overwhelmed. If necessary, ask for clarification.
- Intimidation—Most investigators are very serious about their responsibilities. They usually have years of experience that can cause you to feel anxious when communicating with them. This is understandable. If you are well prepared and aware of the facilities compliance sources, you will feel less intimidated (Fig. 8-2).
- Fear—Fear is a barrier to communication. Fear may be based on potential fines, loss of licensure, or repercussions from your manager. If your health care setting is up to date and follows all regulations, fear should not be a factor.
- Pressure from the manager—Managers often feel the pressure from their superiors, which trickles down to everyone. A comment such as, "Don't mess this up," can create stress and become a barrier to effective communication.

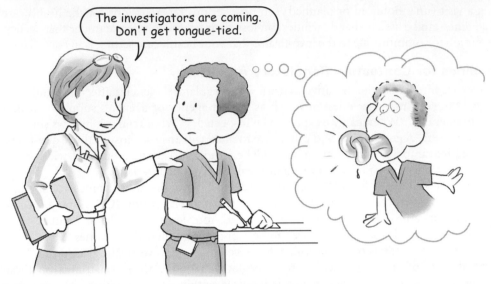

The investigators are coming. Don't get tongue-tied.

Figure 8-2

- "Going against the staff"—During your career, there may be times or situations that make you feel the need to report an incident without your manager's approval. For example, you may feel the health care setting is overbilling for claims, conducting Medicare fraud, or writing illegal prescriptions. No matter what the situation, follow your own ethical standards and always work within the law.

All of these challenges can be difficult to overcome. However, you will be able to overcome them using these tips.

Practical Tips

Use the acronym **AGENCY.**

Answer. Answer the investigator's questions in a professional, nonhostile manner. For example, do not make a comment such as, "Of course we follow all your rules"; instead, calmly and politely say, "We follow all of the regulations within your guidelines."

Give only the appropriate data or information. Give investigators the information they need, but do not offer additional information or data that are not requested. Let investigators lead the investigation.

Encourage open dialogue. Offer your assistance and show your enthusiasm for helping. For example, you may say, "If you have any questions, please let me know. I will be in the next room." This statement shows your cooperative spirit and opens the communication line.

Never hide or conceal any information. Hiding or concealing information can be perceived as a criminal act and you can be held responsible for your actions. If the investigator is looking for certain information, and you know that it's being concealed, do not participate in concealing its existence.

Confidentiality. Know what information must be released and to whom. For example, a patient diagnosed with tuberculosis must be reported to your state's public health department, even if the patient does not want it reported. Before you give investigators patient information, you need to know what agency they represent and what parts of the chart they are allowed access to. For example, an investigator may have access to the chest x-ray report but not to the patient's HIV status. Give only the necessary information. Also, remember to follow the HIPAA regulations.

Your attention: It is important that you communicate to investigators that they have your full attention and participation. For example, comments such as, "Yeah, I'll get that for you in a minute," does not communicate professionalism or respect.

- Know the regulations and stay abreast of them. It is easier to stay current than it is to play catch-up. Ask the investigator "What changes can we expect to see in the next few years?"
- Never offer an investigator a bribe.
- Federal and state agency investigators will always have an official identification badge. Ask to see the badge. Ask for credentials before releasing any information. Some health care settings issue temporary badges for investigators to wear during their visit. If you are assigned to wear a badge, make sure you have it on and it is visible. Badges communicate professionalism and credibility.

Table 8-4 suggests phrases to use—and to avoid—when speaking with a regulatory agency investigator.

Communicating Referral Information

Common Types of Referrals

Patients are often referred to specialists for specific health care issues. A **referral** is a formal contract between two or more health care team members to provide services to a patient. Patients can be referred to specialties, such as those listed in Box 8-1. Other common referrals include home care agencies, social services, and various financial support services.

Table 8-4   Dos and Don'ts for Speaking with Regulatory Agency Investigators

THESE PHRASES PROMOTE COMMUNICATION AND DIALOGUE. DO USE THESE PHRASES:

"Can I answer any questions for you?"
"If you need me I'll be in my office."
"I think you can find everything you need in here."
"That's a good idea. We will try that here."
"Thank you for your suggestions."

THESE PHRASES HINDER COMMUNICATION AND HALT DIALOGUE. DON'T USE THESE PHRASES:

"That's a dumb rule."
"So, what are you looking for?"
"Hurry up."
"There is nothing wrong here"
"We do it our own way."

Physicians often speak to other physicians about specific care issues. For example, an internist may refer a patient to a cardiologist for evaluation and management of the patient's cardiac pathologies. The cardiologist will then treat the patient for his heart problems and the internist will continue to treat the patient's other conditions.

A consultation is different. In a **consultation**, the patient goes to a specialist for an evaluation. Then, the consultant recommends a treatment plan to the primary care doctor. The patient's primary doctor will then treat the condition.

Referrals and consultations are made after discussing the problem with the patient. The patient has the right to accept or refuse another's professional services. For example, the physician may choose to refer the patient to a home care agency for home health aide services but the patient can refuse the service. However, there are exceptions to this rule. If the physician or other health care provider feels the patient or family member needs the services from a protective service agency, the patient or caregiver cannot refuse these services without a court order.

Guidelines for Referrals

You will be involved with assisting the physician in making referrals. Referrals begin with a physician's order. In the order, the physician will communicate to you the following information:

- Type of services needed
- Date services should begin
- Duration of service or goals of the service
- Specific instructions. For example, the physician may refer a patient to a physical therapist for crutch-walking education but may specify the patient is to be "non–weight-bearing for 3 weeks then begin progressive weight-bearing as tolerated."

Depending on the health care facility where you work, there may be "standing orders" allowing you to make certain referrals. For example, a standing order may state, "Refer new patient with type II diabetes to a diabetes educator for glucose monitoring instruction." In this case, the order is already written and you may begin the referral process without consulting the physician.

Follow all HIPAA regulations and make sure the patient has signed a release form. The HIPAA release information sheet should include the patient's name, date, signatures, and any specific guidelines regarding who can and cannot be given patient information (see the Legal Eagle box).

 LEGAL EAGLE

The Health Insurance Portability and Accountability Act (HIPAA) of 1996 is a federal law aimed at protecting individuals' private information. Any information that can identify the patient is protected. This includes the patient's name, address, telephone number, date of birth, and Social Security number. Violations, even accidental, can result in large fines. Knowingly releasing patient information without proper authorization can result in fines against individual providers and institutions.

After the order is written and the HIPAA release form is completed, the referral request can be made. Either an oral or a written report should then be sent to the appropriate agency. If a written report is done, use the appropriate agency form. Print the information neatly. Watch your spelling. Attach any documents as necessary. Written referrals are generally faxed to the agency. It is important to follow-up on written referrals to be sure they were obtained and to determine the progress of the referral.

Practical Tips

Use the acronym **CONSULT.**

Clarify: Clarify terms that you do not understand before making the call. For example, if the physician wrote, "PT to help with gait training," you should know that PT refers to a physical therapist and understand the basics of the term "gait training." Clarify to which agency the referral is to be made. And finally, clarify that the referral agency can assist you with this case before you start to give a lengthy report, only to find that the agency does not offer those services or they cannot meet your time constraints. For example, you may say, "Hello, This is Dr. Robert's office calling with a referral for a patient who needs a physical therapist for gait training in her home. Is this a case that you could help us with?"

Objective data: Give the agency the appropriate demographic data such as the patient's name, age, sex, address, and phone number and then the objective data stating the reason for the referral. For example, "Mrs. Santelgo, 87-year-old female, had a fractured ankle 2 weeks ago and needs a home physical therapist to help her."

Necessary past history: Give the agency the patient's pertinent past medical or surgical history. For example, "She has insulin-dependent diabetes and has a short leg cast on her left leg." It is not necessary to list past surgeries or medical conditions unless they affect the plan of care. Additional information regarding past surgeries or medical conditions (i.e., appendectomy, 1974) can be sent on the referral form.

Symptoms/signs: Provide the agency with a list of the specific symptoms or signs the patient is experiencing in relation to the referral need. For example "Her toes on the left foot are ecchymotic but they are warm and have good capillary refill. She becomes short of breath with minimal exertion."

Unusual circumstances: You should alert the agency to any situations or circumstances that would or could hinder its ability to care for this patient. For example, "She has three big dogs and eight cats." This information is relevant for a home care agency to know so they can select an appropriate physical therapist that is not afraid of dogs or allergic to cats. However, this information would *not* be necessary to communicate if you were calling an outpatient physical therapy department and the patient was going to be seen inside their facility for gait training.

Looking: Explain in detail what services the patient is looking to obtain. Include any information about time constraints. For example, "She needs to have the physical therapist come in the afternoon. She goes to the outpatient clinic in the mornings for her chemotherapy. She is home by 1 p.m."

Time: Explain to the referring agency when you want or need the services to start. For example, "The doctor would like the services to start this week. Is this possible?" If the agency personnel cannot reasonably guarantee the services, you need to communicate that to the physician so other arrangements can be made.

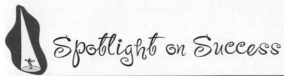

Creating a good working relationship with various referral agencies can be advantageous to your career and your advancement. Many health job opportunities are never advertised. They are spread through networking. Networking grows by communicating with your colleagues inside your office and outside your setting. Every time that you speak with a referral agency, think of it as a networking opportunity. You never know when an exciting job will arise. Being in the right place, at the right time, and having the right friends can make it happen.

Create good networking skills by open and honest communication with referral agencies (see Spotlight on Success box). Do not hide or conceal issues regarding the patient. Do not exaggerate the patient's conditions. Never gossip. Provide only the facts in a professional, nonjudgmental manner.

COMMUNICATING WHEN YOU ARE IN CHARGE

Communication Challenges

There are numerous challenges to being in charge. You are no longer "one of the gang." Usually, your first management position will be in a middle management or supervisory role. This means that you will have a title such as "assistant office manager" or "assistant clinical coordinator" and will be given some administrative duties but will have limited power to change or revamp existing rules.

Peer competition may also exist. A newly hired manager often receives this promotion after a selection process from which other coworkers who had applied were excluded. You may feel challenged by those who also wanted the position. To receive their respect, you need to communicate that you respect them and welcome their support.

Practical Tips

One of the most important rules in communicating from a position of authority is to know your department, recognize the problem areas, and understand why they exist. Get to know your coworkers. It is very difficult to communicate effectively when you lack background information.

Always communicate positive and encouraging information. Actively listen to what your coworkers tell you; think before you speak.

Use the acronym **BOSS**.

Behavior: Explain the behavior that *you* have noticed. Do not accuse or place blame. For example, state " *I* have noticed that the quality controls are not being done on a regular basis."

Objective: Provide the staff with objective findings, not subjective comments. For example, "According to this sheet, *we* are only 75% compliant." Use the word "we" to show that this is a team problem, not an individual's problem.

Spreads: Explain how this spreads and affects other people, patients, or staff. For example, "It is important that *we* are compliant with these checks for the safety of our patients, and it is a regulatory requirement."

Suggest/search: Provide some suggestions for resolving the problem or ask your staff for ideas. For example, " *I* have two ideas on how *we* can improve this. *We* could rotate the responsibility to different times or I could assign a person to do it. Does anyone have any other suggestions?" Another possible sentence would be "*We* haven't had this issue before; what has changed to cause it?" By searching for the root of the problem, you will be able to resolve the problem more quickly and easily.

Notice the words "I" and "we" are used. Avoid the word "you". For example, avoid saying "You are not doing the quality checks." As soon as you use the word "you," the listener assumes a defensive mode and a communication barrier rises.

- Offer positive reinforcement. For example, "Last week we reached 100% compliance. Great job everyone." Praise coworkers as often as possible. This increases self-esteem and has been proven to increase work output.

- Try to communicate that we need to overcome these "challenges." Avoid using the word "problems." For example, it is better to say, "We have a staffing challenge ahead of us" rather than saying "We have a staffing problem." The word "problem" creates a negative image.

- Use phrases such as, "We have an opportunity to improve." The word "improve" projects a positive image and outlook.

The Art of Delegation

As the manager, you will need to delegate certain projects. **Delegating** is the process of carefully assigning a project or task to someone who you feel is competent to complete the task within a given time. Before you can safely delegate any task, you must know your staff's ability and **competency** level. Competency means that the staff person has been trained and successfully passed an evaluation for a given task. You need to know who your staff members are and what they can do safely. Ask yourself "What is this person's individual competency level?" Competency levels vary based on staff experiences, job titles, and educational background. After determining that someone is competent, decide a reasonable timeframe for the project to be completed. Once you have decided who is responsible for the task and you decide when the task needs to be completed, you can then communicate that information to your staff member. You will not be effective at delegating if you say, "I need someone to do this project. It should be done soon."

To delegate projects and have your staff complete them requires that you be an effective leader and that you can communicate in a positive manner. Here are other points to help you get started:

- Energize your staff
- Encourage your staff to be independent thinkers and workers
- Encourage your staff to self-manage
- Encourage your staff to brainstorm ideas

When you are ready to delegate, remember the power of the Ps: Don't pressure, preach, or punish: Instead praise, persuade, and promote.

Avoid phrases such as "calm down." Instead you may say, "I see you are upset, let's talk about what is going on." Let the other person talk while you actively listen. Listen between the lines. Allow periods of silence. Recap conversations, such as, "If I understand correctly, this is the problem." Then, rephrase the problem. Ask for resolution ideas. This helps your team feel part of the solution rather than part of the problem.

Communicating Support and Compassion

When you are in charge, occasionally you will be confronted with staff's personal problems. Examples of personal problems are death of family members, financial problems, or divorces. It is easy to become absorbed in such problems, but you need to keep everything in perspective. When you are in charge, you need to communicate empathy and not sympathy. Chapter 1 discusses these terms with a patient focus. Below you will find some additional information about applying these skills when you are in charge.

Empathy is understanding and caring about another person's problem. It requires that you suspend judgment or avoid jumping to conclusions. With empathy, you must try to walk in another person's shoes for the moment. It does not mean that you need to agree, but that you emotionally understand their feelings. Once you understand the situation, then you can give support and encouragement. Here are some phrases that promote empathy, "Let's talk about what is happening," "Tell me about your situation." Use the power of silence to let the other person tell you what is happening. Give the conversation your full attention and work toward a thorough understanding.

Sympathy means that you feel the same emotions the other person feels. If someone is sad, you feel sad; if someone feels anxious, you feel anxious. If you sympathize with every staff member's problems, you will be unable to work as a manager effectively. You need to be able to understand the problem and then consider how it will impact the team.

Consider the following situation:

Manager #1: "I understand that you are going through a divorce; let's talk about how we can meet your needs and the needs of the department."

Manager #2: "I am sorry that you are going through a divorce. You must be very upset. Let me know what I can do to help."

Which statement makes a bigger impact?

Manager #1 communicates empathy. She demonstrates that she understands the problem and is working to resolve it as it pertains to the workplace. Manager #2 communicates sympathy but sounds insincere and does not work towards a solution.

Communicating in the health care setting requires that you openly and honestly communicate with patients and team members. There will be occasional communication barriers, but with the use of various acronyms, you will get your points across. Take a moment to think before you speak and it will make all the difference in communicating in the workplace.

Taking the Chapter to Work

Now, let's meet Sue and Ramona and see how they have applied this chapter information in the workplace.

Sue is working in a pediatrician's office. She has been asked to come to a case conference regarding the Flash family. The Flash family consists of a single mother with four children. The father of two of the children is in jail and the paternity of the other children is unclear. The pediatrician begins the case conference by asking Sue to report on the number of appointments Ms. Flash has cancelled. Sue communicates the information and mentions that Ms. Flash has told her "she does not have a car and transportation is a problem." A social worker mentions that the Flash family is eligible for free bus passes to doctor's appointments. The members discuss the bus pass policy and agree that this is a good solution. The pediatrician directs the social worker to get the passes and have them mailed to Ms. Flash. Then, the pediatrician asks Sue to communicate the bus pass information to Ms. Flash. Sue's ability to communicate the facts in an organized manner allows the team to identify and correct a problem. This improves patient care.

Ramona is working at Mayhew's Obstetrical and Gynecology Office. The receptionist calls her and states that a young woman has just arrived and is bleeding. Ramona talks to the woman and determines that she is 28 weeks' pregnant and started vaginally bleeding about 20 minutes ago. Ramona recognizes this is an emergent situation and contacts the physician STAT. The physician returns the page and Ramona communicates the patient information in a calm, concise manner. The physician tells Ramona that she is in the office elevator and will be there in a moment. Ramona tells the patient that the doctor is coming and offers her reassurance. The physician exams the patient and decides to have her transported to the hospital via an ambulance. Ramona calls for the ambulance and communicates with the dispatcher. Then, Ramona tells the receptionist to direct the ambulance personnel into the appropriate examination room. Ramona and the physician communicate the patient information to the ambulance technicians. Lastly, Ramona calls the patient's spouse and alerts him to the situation. She communicates with the spouse in a calm manner and offers reassurance.

This emergent event was handled smoothly because Ramona communicated with the receptionist, physician, patient, ambulance dispatcher, and technicians. She also took the time to talk with the patient's spouse. Ramona's communication skills improved patient care.

Beyond the Classroom Exercises

Your Assignment Board

The following exercises will help you use your new knowledge. Place a check mark beside the assignments that your instructor has given you. When you have completed the assignment, place a check mark in the completed column.

		Assigned	*Completed*
Checking Your Comprehension	(Textbook)	❏	❏
Expanding Critical Thinking	(Textbook)	❏	❏
Communication Surfer Exercises	(Textbook and Internet)	❏	❏
Communication Branch #11	(CD-ROM)	❏	❏
Communication Branch #12	(CD-ROM)	❏	❏
Voice Mail Message #8	(CD-ROM)	❏	❏

Checking Your Comprehension

Write a brief answer to each of the following assignments.
1. Define the term *professional etiquette*. Give three examples of proper etiquette when working in a health care setting.
2. List three goals of interdisciplinary communication.
3. Define the terms *emergent, urgent,* and *nonurgent*. Give an example of when to contact a physician for each type.
4. What acronym can help you communicate with your coworkers? Explain each letter.
5. What acronym can help you communicate with a physician? Explain each letter.
6. Name five regulatory agencies and explain their role in the health care setting.
7. Define the term *delegate*.

Expanding Critical Thinking

1. Envision yourself communicating an important message to each of the five groups covered in this chapter. Write a brief explanation of each problem. Then write a communication dialogue using the appropriate acronym for each group.
2. You suspect that the physician for whom you are working is overbilling Medicare for procedures that are not done. How would you discuss this issue? With whom would you discuss it? What are the legal implications of not reporting Medicare fraud?
3. During your job orientation, you notice that your new employer is using an outdated blood pathogen standard. How would you go about discussing this with her? What Internet website would you use to download current blood-borne pathogen standards? What key words could you use on a search engine?
4. Think about your best friend. Could you work effectively with her or him? Why or why not? Assume that you have developed a conflict working together. How would you feel about communicating this problem? What steps can you take to increase your comfort level?
5. How do you feel about communicating with physicians? Do you feel intimidated? What steps can you take to improve your comfort level?

Communication Surfer Exercises

1. Find the JCAHO Internet site. Locate and print five sample standards. Explain the intent of these standards in your own words. What is JCAHO's mission?
2. Find your state's Department of Health Internet site. Which communicable diseases need to be reported? What is the time for reporting? How should you report these conditions?
3. Find the U.S. Food and Drug Administration Internet site. How would you communicate with them regarding a defective medical device? What are the guidelines for reporting defective medical devices?
4. Find the Occupational Safety Health Administration Internet site. What is OSHA's mission? What is the process to report a workplace injury?

9

COMMUNICATING TO GET THE JOB YOU WANT: FOUR KEY TOOLS

LEARNING OBJECTIVES

Upon successfully completing this chapter, you will be able to:

- Describe the components of a resume.
- List 10 key action words that can strengthen a resume.
- Describe eight practical tips for writing your resume.
- State 10 commonly asked interview questions and give possible personal responses.
- Describe five practical tips for surviving a job interview.
- Explain the purpose for writing a thank-you letter.
- Write a resume, cover letter, and thank-you letter.

KEY TERMS

Chronological	Functional	Objective
Cover letter	Interview	Resume
Demographics	Multitask	Template

Test Your Communication **IQ**

Before reading this chapter, complete this short self-assessment test. Decide which statements are true and which are false.

1. The purpose of a resume is to tell prospective employers everything about you and your life.
2. If you were terminated by an employer, you should include that position on your resume.
3. It is a good idea to exaggerate your accomplishments when writing a resume.
4. Calligraphy or other fancy fonts should be used on a resume.
5. A cover letter is a powerful marketing tool to sell yourself.
6. You should never answer any interviewer's questions about your marital status.
7. You should not ask questions during the interview process because the purpose of the interview is for the interviewer to get to know you and learn about your skills.

Results

Statements two and five are true; all the other statements are false. How did you do? Read the chapter to find more information on these topics.

COMMUNICATION TOOL NUMBER ONE: THE RESUME

A good first impression is essential to getting your dream job. Your **resume** is often the first impression a prospective employer has of you. A resume is a factual document that outlines your professional and academic experiences. Make it count!

There are numerous formats for writing a resume. The two most common are functional and chronological. Each style has similar components but they appear in a different sequence. First, lets examine the components of a resume and then discuss formatting.

Components of a Resume

A standard resume should consist of five components:
- Demographics
- Objective
- Educational experiences
- Work experiences
- Awards, certifications, or licenses

Here is a closer look at each of these items.

Demographics

Demographics refers to your personal identification information. At minimum, it should include your name, address, and telephone number. Your full legal name is given on the top line. Do not abbreviate your first name. For example, write Jessica Stricker and not J. Stricker. Your friends may call you "Jes" but your legal name is Jessica and therefore it should be written as such. A middle name should be included if you routinely use it. It is acceptable to use only your middle initial. For example, write Jessica E. Stricker, if you routinely use E. for formal documents. Following your name, attach any professional designations that you have obtained. For example: C.M.A., R.M.A., L.P.N., R.N., P.T., C.N.A., or E.M.T. If you include any such designations, be sure to include a copy of the certification/license with your resume.

Your address should include the street name and number, town or city, state and zip code. Your street number and name is listed on a line by itself. If you are using a post office box, it is recommended that you include your street address as well. On the third line, include the town or city followed by a comma and then the state. Write out the whole name of the state. Do not use abbreviations. Abbreviations do not portray a professional image. Place a comma after the state, and type the zip code.

Your home telephone number should appear on the next line. Include the area code in parenthesis followed by the number. It is acceptable to use either dashes (-) or periods between the numbers. For example, you could write your telephone number as (888)555-3333 or 888.555.3333. It is not recommended to include cell phone numbers on your resume.

If you have an e-mail address, it can be included on the line below the telephone number. Caution: if you list an e-mail address as a communication line, check for messages at least once a day and respond promptly. Be sure that your e-mail address is appropriate. An e-mail address such as badgirls@something.net is not professional and should not be used.

Objective

An **objective** is a statement of your goals or intentions. It should be precise, focused, and brief. Keep your objective statement to one or two sentences. The purpose of the objective is to let prospective employers know what you are looking for in a job. Here are some examples of good objectives:

- To find a (nursing, medical assisting) position that allows me to work in a medical setting caring for sick children.
- To find a challenging and fast-paced position as a (nurse, therapist, medical assistant) in an acute care setting.

  Here are some bad examples:
- I want a job in the medical field.
- I am looking for a high paying job in the medical field in New York City.

Your objective statement should be changed to reflect the type of job for which you are applying. For example, "to find a challenging and fast-paced position as a medical assistant in an acute care setting" is a good objective only if you are applying to an acute care setting. If you are applying to an outpatient clinic, you should change the objective to say: "to find a challenging and fast-paced position as a medical assistant in an outpatient clinic."

Educational Experience

This section covers your educational experiences in a reverse chronological order. Provide the full name of the school with no abbreviations, including the city and state. A street address is not needed. If you are a graduate, list the degree that you were awarded. Include the date that you graduated. If you are still a student, list the year that you enrolled, for example write "2004–present."

List only post-secondary educational experiences. You do not need to list your high school graduation. Do not list continuing educational courses that you have attended. For example, if you attended a special seminar on pediatric care, it should not be listed in this section. Make a chronological list of special continuing educational seminars and either send it with your resume or bring it to the interview. Make sure that the seminars are relevant and keep the list to one page only. Be sure to include the dates of attendance.

Work Experience

This section of your resume lists your employment history. Start with your job title, followed by the company's name, and city and state. A street address is not necessary. Include the dates, for example, "June 2003–present." It is not necessary to add the day, just the month and year. You can either bullet or write two or three short sentences describing your responsibilities. Bullets alert the reader to pay attention. Keep the list of your responsibilities to a maximum of five. Highlight your key responsibilities. Every job has numerous subjobs, but ask yourself "What do I want to communicate about this job?" "Why will this previous job make me the best candidate to get this new job?" Make each entry or bullet count. Here are some things that you should *not* do:

- Do not list your salary.
- Do not include your supervisor's name.
- Do not list or explain why you left a position.
- Do not overstate your accomplishments. For example, you would not want to say, "Developed, wrote, and published new patient education materials," unless you actually single-handedly did these three things. Perhaps you were on the committee that revamped patient education material, in which case a better bullet would be, "Participated in patient education committee and helped to recreate and update new patient education materials."

Awards/Certifications/Licenses

The final component of a resume is the list of your awards, certifications, and licenses (see Legal Eagle box). They should be pertinent to the job for which you are applying. As a new graduate, it may be difficult to have a lengthy list. Here are some things to remember:

- All health care employers like to see "Cardiopulmonary Resuscitation" certifications. You can become CPR certified through either the American Heart Association or American Red Cross. Generally, it is a 6- to 8-hour course. Even if it is not a job requirement, it shows that you took the initiative to complete the course.
- If you have just graduated and are pending licensure or certification results, indicate the month and year that you took the examination and the name of the licensure examination and accrediting agency. For example: "Pending results of Licensed Practical Nurse examination for State of Connecticut, June 2005."

 LEGAL EAGLE

It is illegal to tamper with a state-issued professional license. Claiming that you have a "license" as a nurse, paramedic, or other health care professional for which you do *not* is a criminal offense. This could result in imprisonment and fines. It may later bar you from applying for that license. It is also illegal to falsify the information supplied on your license application. It could result in your being barred from having your license renewed.

- Before being eligible to sit for a certification examination, you often are required to complete a certain number of clinical hours. In this case, communicate that by writing, "Plan to take (add the name) Certification Examination in June 2005. Completed 50 of the 100 hours of clinical experience required."

Practical Tips for Creating a Resume

There are many resources for building a resume. The CD-ROM included in this book has a resume **template**. A template is an outline that allows you to enter key information and create a document. Here are some general rules about creating a resume:
- Keep your resume to one page if possible; two is considered maximum.
- Emphasize things that you have achieved or accomplished but do not exaggerate or embellish the facts.
- Do not mention personal information (such as age, sex, marital status).
- Select an appropriate format to highlight your talents.

Various Internet sites offer resume building and critiquing, although a charge is usually associated with these services. You can find resume builders in your local telephone book. Before spending money on a professional resume writer, contact your school's guidance or placement office. Most schools also offer resume writing free of charge or for a nominal fee. Spending extra time and attention to create your resume will communicate professionalism and help you get the job you desire.

Resume Formats

As mentioned above, there are numerous formats for writing a resume. Be aware that the formats used and the preferred methods change periodically. In the medical community, the two most common formats are chronological and functional.

A **chronological** resume (Fig. 9-1) is the most commonly used. This format works best for people who have extensive work experience but have been out of school for a while or have a limited educational background. The chronological resume focuses on your progressive work experiences. Following is the order of a chronological resume:
1. Work experiences—List your most recent position and work backwards. Describe your job experiences and responsibilities.
2. Educational experiences
3. Awards/certifications/licenses

A **functional** resume (Fig. 9-2) lists your skills or accomplishments in categories. This resume is good for people with limited work experiences, new graduates, or people returning to the work force. The focus of a functional resume is on the skills you have and not when or where you obtained these skills. Following is the order of a functional resume:
1. Accomplishments or competencies are listed first. They can be broken into various categories, such as clinical skills, administrative skills, and laboratory skills. Dates or employment records are not assigned to the skill.
2. Employment experiences: List the most recent first and work backwards. List only the dates, job title, and name of the facility.
3. Educational experiences
4. List any awards/certifications/licensures

Ruby Dunham
9365 Caesar Creek Road
Mytown, OH 45458
(937) 555-1899

Experience:

2004-present: Medical Transcriptionist, Community Hospital,
Mytown OH

· Transcribe 55 wpm
· Specialist in medical terminology
· Excellent attendance record
· Detail oriented
· Increased personal productivity each quarter

2003-2004: Secretary, State University School of Medicine,
Mytown, OH

· Coordinated schedules of four full-time professors
· Maintained office supply and assistant budget
· Created scheduling guidelines for department
· Developed excellent written communication skills
· Familiar with a variety of office machines

2001-2003: Shift manager, Burger World, Mytown,OH

· Managed 10 employees, including hiring, training, evaluating,
  and firing
· Developed excellent oral commuicaton skills and team player
  concept
· Improved inventory supply techniques, reducing losses by 10%
· Maintained cleanliness standards highest in chain
· Developed customer-focused service goals for store

Education:

· 2004: A.S. in Medical Assisting, Community College, Mytown, OH

Figure 9-1
Chronological resume.

Composing

Composing simply means to write. Start by gathering all the necessary information. Check your dates for accuracy. Select your format (chronological or functional). If you are not using a template, select a word processing program. Select an appropriate font and size. The font should be clear and easy to read. Avoid elaborate or calligraphy style fonts.

When writing a resume, choose your words carefully. Select words that demonstrate action. Remember: the purpose of a resume is to communicate your accomplishments to a prospective employer. Box 9-1 lists some sample action words.

Max Bryan
1234 Rolling View Court
Mytown, OH 45458
(937) 555-1899

OBJECTIVE

· An entry-level position in medical assisting, with the opportunity to utilize and refine skills and training

ACCOMPLISHMENTS

· Tutored students in medical assisting and 12-lead EKG courses
   (received excellent evaluations and positive results)
· Certified Medical Assistant, active member of local AAMA
· Experienced in MS Office programs
· Consistent "excellent" ratings in clinical externships

STRENGTHS

· Possess excellent interpersonal and communication skills
· Demonstrate consistent positive attitude and high energy
· Caring and compassionate
· Responsible, self-motivated, precise in work
· Experienced in customer-focused service

EMPLOYMENT

· 2003-present: Tutor, Community College, Mytown, OH
· Waiter, Scott's Place, Mytown, OH

EDUCATION

· 2004: A.S. in Medical Assisting, Community College, Mytown, OH
   Dean's list senior year, cumulative GPA 3.5

COMMUNITY ACTIVITIES

· 2001-present: Organized, recruited, and trained 20 others for church
   hand bell choir, direct weekly practices and monthly performances
· 2002-present: Teach community CPR twice yearly to high school
   students
· Vice-President Student Government, Community College, Mytown,
   OH. Recruited members, organized fund-raisers, campaigned
   successfully for policy changes

Figure 9-2
Functional resume.

Editing

Editing is perhaps the most crucial step. Check, double-check, and triple-check your resume. Editing uncovers errors in punctuation and spelling, misused words, and poor grammar. Even one misspelled word can be disastrous. Documents with grammatical errors do not portray a positive, professional image. They indicate that you do not pay attention to detail

Box **9-1**   **Action Words**

These words command respect and demonstrate accomplishments:

Achieved	Identified
Applied	Operated
Conducted	Organized
Completed	Oriented (new staff)
Constructed	Performed
Developed	Prepared
Directed	Processed
Educated/taught	Scheduled
Handled	Solved
Generated	

and that your work habits may be sloppy. Check dates for accuracy. Be sure that the information is factually correct.

Honesty

It might seem innocent to tweak the facts or to embellish the truth, but it is a risk that can have serious repercussions. False information on a resume or an application can be grounds for later termination. State only the facts. It is equally as bad to "leave out" information on a resume. For example, let's say that you were fired from Dr. Jones' office. Should you still list Dr. Jones under the section "work experience?" Yes, you should. State the dates you were employed. Be prepared to answer questions during the interview as to why you left the office.

Printing Suggestions

Print your resume on either white or off-white paper. Use a good-quality paper (20 or 24 pound). Black ink is preferred. Never use colors for either print or paper. Make sure that your printer cartridge is new and full. After printing the resume, examine it for smudging or streaking. Reprint it as needed.

COMMUNICATION TOOL NUMBER TWO: THE COVER LETTER

A **cover letter** is a formal document that introduces your resume. The cover letter should catch the interest of prospective employers so that they will want to read your resume. Think of a cover letter as a marketing tool to sell yourself. Keep in mind that this prospective employer has advertised for a position and has probably received many other resumes. You need to communicate why your resume should float to the top of the pile. A resume without a cover letter is unprofessional and indicates lack of follow-through.

Components of a Cover Letter

A cover letter (Fig. 9-3) should have the appropriate demographic information, three paragraphs, and a closing. Let's look at each of these components:

Demographics

This should match your resume demographics. Follow the same guidelines and double-check the information for accuracy. Ask yourself: Did I use my legal name? Is my middle initial used, and if so I did I use it on my resume? Did I type my correct address? Did I include my street number and apartment or unit number? Did I remember to type the town, city, state, and zip code? Did I transpose any of my telephone numbers? These may seem like little mistakes but they communicate to the reader that you are careless and do not pay attention to detail.

Introductory Paragraph

This paragraph should consist of three or four sentences. Begin by stating how you found out about this position. For example, "I read your advertisement in the *Hartford Courant* on Sunday, February 2, 2005 for a (use the *exact* wording in the advertisement)." Your second sentence should indicate that you know something about the clinic or medical setting. For example, "I am familiar with the services that your clinic offers." Or "I am aware of Doctor Miranda's excellent reputation as a hand surgeon." The third sentence should draw a conclusion that you meet the needs of the advertisement. Here is an example of a good third sentence, "I have the clinical skills and background needed for this position."

Body of the Letter

This should consist of one paragraph that communicates in a "nut shell" why your skills and background meet the needs of this particular job. Reread the advertisement. Use many of those exact words or phrases in this paragraph. If the advertisement says, "Must be familiar with XYZ software program," then you should state, "I have used XYZ software and I am comfortable with its applications." If the ad stated, "Must be able to perform phlebotomy," then you need to communicate that you are proficient in phlebotomy.

If the advertisement states that you "Must be able to start IVs," and you cannot start IVs then you need to ask yourself "is this the right job for me?" However, suppose you can start IVs but have not practiced them lately; be honest and say, "I learned to start IVs during my clinical rotation in the hospital. I am comfortable with the skill and look forward to an opportunity to enhance my competency."

Concluding Paragraph

The purpose of this paragraph is to encourage the prospective employer to call you for an interview. You want to communicate enthusiasm for obtaining an interview and excitement about the position. This paragraph should contain two or three sentences. An example of a good sentence would be, "I would appreciate the opportunity to meet with you and discuss how my clinical skills would benefit your clinic." End with a sentence such as, "I look forward to hearing from you."

Type an appropriate closing, such as "Sincerely." Leave at least three spaces and type your complete name exactly as it appears on the top of the letter. Sign the letter in the space between the closing and your typed name.

Ann Marie Brown

123 Walnut Street, Apt. 4-C

Williamsburg, Connecticut 12345

888.333.5555

abrown01@email.com

January 17, 2005

Rebecca Ames, RN

Nurse Manager

Women's Health Clinic

123 Main Street

Middletown, Connecticut 01234

Dear Ms. Ames:

I am responding to your advertisement in the *Hometown Journal* on Sunday, April 29th for a Medical Assistant for the Women's Health Clinic. I recently read in the paper about the clinic's exciting new expansion plans. I feel that my experience and enthusiasm would be a benefit to the clinic.

I graduated from the Health Care Institute in December 2003. During my externship, I worked at a women's clinic in Hartford and was subsequently hired by them to fill a temporary vacancy. I am very comfortable performing various administrative duties, including the use of the Medi-Plus computer system.

I look forward to an opportunity to meet with you to discuss this position. Thank you for considering me for the Medical Assistant position at the Women's Health Clinic.

Sincerely,

Ann Marie Brown

Figure 9-3
Cover letter.

Practical Tips for Writing a Cover Letter

In addition to the above-mentioned steps, the following are some practical tips for writing a cover letter:

- Before you type the letter, know to whom it should be addressed. Make sure you have the individual's title correct and the spelling correct.
- Mistakes are not acceptable. Poor spelling, punctuation, and grammar will reflect poorly on you.
- Print a copy of your resume and proofread it. It often helps to print it, leave it for awhile, and then come back to it. Reread it with a fresh look. Ask a friend to proofread it.
- Make the corrections, save the document, and print a final copy. Look at the copy for smudge marks.
- Sign your name neatly. Use either a blue or black pen.
- Place the cover letter on top of the resume, and fold them neatly into thirds. Make the crease solid.
- Type the envelope. Handwritten envelopes do not communicate professionalism.

Once you send out the resume and cover letter, be prepared for telephone calls. Let family members know that you are expecting important calls. Have a message pad and pen at the telephone. Make sure that your answering machine message has a pleasant and mature message. The voice on the message should be clear. Loud background music is not appropriate. An example of an appropriate message would be " Hi. This is Tonya. I am not available to take your call at this moment. Please leave your name, phone number, and message after the beep. I will return your call as soon as possible." Check for messages regularly and return calls promptly.

COMMUNICATION TOOL NUMBER THREE: THE INTERVIEW

Commonly Asked Interview Questions and the Answers

Congratulations, you have secured a job **interview**. An interview is a two-way discussion between a potential employee and an employer. This is your one chance to make a good and lasting impression on your prospective employer. Preparation is key. Many standard questions are asked during a job interview. In the next few paragraphs, some of the most commonly asked questions are discussed, along with sample responses. These are only suggested responses. Add information that is unique to you and that displays your qualities and characteristics. Be sure to emphasize your strengths and accomplishments.

It is best to rehearse answering these questions in front of a mirror or by asking a friend to role-play an interview. Try to keep your answers short and concise. Do not give long, drawn-out answers or deviate from the question being asked. Avoid rambling. But, by the same token, avoid single word answers such as "yes" or "no."

Personal Questions

Most interviewers start the interview by asking you personal questions. This helps them get to know you on a personal level. Quite often the first question will be something like, "Tell me something about yourself." Describe yourself using positive action words. For example "I am a very motivated person." "I enjoy working with people." Your response should be about 1 to 2 minutes long. Do not go into your personal hobbies or interests. These are some other common personal style questions.

- *How would you define success?* A good response would be, "I define success as being able to achieve my highest potential through working hard and striving to be the best person that I can be."

- *What is your greatest accomplishment?* The interviewer is looking for one solid example of an accomplishment. A good response would be, "My greatest accomplishment was graduating from (your school's name). I accomplished this through hard work and learned many valuable lessons."

- *How would you describe your personality?* Use a dictionary or thesaurus and plan your answer. Some possible words or phrases could be team player, honest, sensitive, self-motivated, punctual, and flexible. Make sure that your voice sounds strong and secure. Often our self-esteem does not allow us to boast about our positive traits, but you need to be able to communicate some positive aspects such as "I am a good role model" or "I am a very dedicated person."

- *What are your short- and long-term goals?* Interviewers like to ask this question to determine where you see yourself in the next 3 months, 6 months, and 5 years. If you state, "I hope to move to Florida next year," the interviewer must consider the cost of orienting an employee for probably just 1 year. A good response would be: "I hope that I will have found a position that challenges me and will remain in that position for the next few years. My long-term goal is to continue taking college courses to obtain my Associates degree."

- *Are you happy with your career choice? If you were to start a new career, what would it be?* A good answer would be: "I am enjoying my career as a (fill in your title). If I were to start a new career, it would be an extension of my current trade." (Then give an example). Be careful making statements such as, "I would be a politician, veterinarian, etc." While you may always wish to become something totally different, it communicates to the interviewer that you are unsure of who you are and what you want.

- *What types of people do you work best with or worse? And why?* Saying something such as "I don't care for bossy people," or "I like laid back people" implies that you are that type of person. We usually prefer people who are like us. A better response would be: "I like people who are self-motivated, independent and enjoy working together." When asked about types of people you would prefer not to work with, avoid the use of the word hate, for example do not say "I hate messy people." Instead remain positive and say, "I prefer not to work with people who are not as well organized as I am."

- *Why did you choose to become a (fill in your job title)?* "I decided to become a (nurse, therapist, medical assistant) because I love to help people. I learned how important it is to be a caring health care worker when I saw my grandmother in the hospital." You can be a little personal with this response, but keep the answer to 1 to 2 minutes.

- *How would your fellow employees describe you?* Interviewers like this question because it gives them an insight into your ability to work with other people. A good answer would be: "They would describe me as a hard worker, organized, fair, fun to be around, flexible." Use only the adjectives that describe you.

Educational Questions

These questions address your educational experiences during your course work. If you have limited work experience, the answers that you give to these questions are crucial. You need to communicate that you have the knowledge and skills that this position requires. Here are some typical questions:

- *What do you know about the position for which you are applying?* You need to communicate to the interviewer that you have a basic understanding of this position. A good response would be "My understanding is that this is a full time LPN position, working nights, on the hospice unit." Then, you should expand on the position by saying something such as, "Hospice nursing is a unique specialty because it focuses on providing end-of-life care to patients and providing support to their families."

- *How do you stay informed professionally?* Be prepared to answer how you obtain continuing education courses. Your best answer is something such as, "I am a member of the (name of your organization) and attend many of the local chapter meetings. I have brought a list of the classes I attended last year. I also subscribe to the (name of the journal or magazine)."

- *I noticed on your transcripts that you failed Microbiology. Tell me about that.* Be honest and say, "Yes, I failed that course, but I took it again last semester and did very well. I find it very difficult to use a microscope." Never say, "The teacher was not fair, it was too hard." Instead be honest, admit your weakness, and then state what you did to make it up.

- *Which class was the hardest? Which was the easiest?* Again, be honest and straight-forward. Do not say, "Pharmacology was the easiest because the teacher just gave out As." Think about the classes you took and the job for which you are applying. If you were applying to work with children, a good response could be "My easiest class was Pediatrics because I really enjoyed the topic and loved to read about the various stages of child development."

- *Who was your favorite teacher and why?* Again, be careful. Do not say, "Mrs. Meza because she never gave us any homework." A better response would be, " I liked Mr. Raymond's class because he helped us reach our full potential."

- *Where did you complete your clinical rotations? Tell me about your evaluations.* Have a list of a few of your clinical sites. A response such as, "Umm, I think we did a rotation at ABC clinic," shows that you are not devoted to your career or education. "I did a rotation at Middlesex Hospital. My clinical rotation evaluations were very good. Ms. Brown was my clinical instructor and I have listed her on my references." This last response shows good organizational skills.

Experience Questions

This is your opportunity to flaunt your strengths. Admit to weaknesses, but have a plan in place for improving them. Here are some sample questions about work experiences:

- *Describe your best boss. Worst boss.* This question allows the interviewer to determine if you will be a good match with her. It also gives a lot of information about your work ethics. A good response would be, "My best boss was Ms. Zoey. She was enthusiastic, fair, and easy to talk to." A bad response would be, "My best boss was Ms. Zoey because she allowed us to come into work in scrubs. She didn't care if we punched in or out. We still got paid." This is a bad response because it implies that you are comfortable in an unprofessional atmosphere. A possible answer for the question about worst boss would be, "My worst boss was at the Main Street Clinic. She was not as organized as I would have liked. I like strong organization skills." This statement is honest and sounds positive. Do not say "She didn't know anything" or "She was old and out of touch." These statements are very negative.

- *What were your duties? Did you dislike any of those duties?* Be prepared to promptly list at least six or seven duties. The worst answer you could give would be, "I did a whole bunch of stuff." This answer is unprofessional and portrays a lazy attitude. A better answer would be, "Some of my clinical duties were …. I also performed some administrative duties such as …." Be honest if there was a particular duty or task that you did not like to do, tell the interviewer. If you did not like doing it before, you probably will not like to do it at a new job. For example, you might say "I did not enjoy drawing blood."

- *Tell me about your most challenging patient.* Start by saying something such as, "I have cared for many interesting and challenging patients." Then describe a particular case. Never use the patient's name; remember patient confidentiality. If possible, try to relate it to the job for which you are applying. For example, if you are applying for a position in a pediatrician's office, using a case involving a child would be better than giving a scenario about an elderly woman.
- *Do you like to work alone? Are you a team player?* This can be a tricky question. In most medical settings, you will be expected to be a team player. However, if you are applying to a small clinic that may do research, or a small office such as a podiatrist's office, the interviewer would then want to make sure that you can work alone and independently. If you are applying to large setting, a good response would be: "I am a team player. I enjoy collaborating with my peers." If you are applying to a small physician's office, a good response would be: "I feel comfortable working independently and I am very self-motivated."
- *How often did you meet with your supervisor?* This is a great question that allows the interviewer to find out about your past performance. If you say, "My supervisor called me into the office at least once a week," a red flag will go up in the interviewer's mind. A better answer would be, "During my 3 years at Midstate clinic, I met with my supervisor periodically to discuss work-related issues. For example, we talked about …." Then give positive examples of such communication.
- *How many pay raises did you receive in your last employment?* This question gives the interviewer a good look into your job performance. It would be assumed that if you received an annual pay raise, that your performance was adequate. However, if you state that you have not gotten a pay raise in 3 years, the interviewer may become suspicious. If pay raises were frozen due to budget concerns, be sure to state that.
- *Anticipate questions toward the specialty for which you are applying.* For example, if you are applying to work with pediatrics, anticipate questions about your ability to care for children. Conversely, if you are applying to work for an oncologist, be prepared for questions about your knowledge of caring for cancer patients.

Stress Management Questions

Working as a medical professional is stressful. No matter whether you are working in a clinic, physician's office, or hospital, your job will be stressful. Certain positions and areas have a higher stress level than others. The interviewer must determine your ability to handle stressful situations. You must be able to communicate how well you handle stress. Types of stress that all medical professionals face are busy schedules, multitasking, and handling unpredictable situations. Be ready for questions such as the following:

- *Are you able to multitask?* **Multitask** is a term used by medical professionals who are required to do more than one thing at a time, in various situations, and do them safely. The ability to multitask takes practice and experience. A good answer to this question would be, "I am comfortable with my many skills and I can perform them under pressure."
- *Are you comfortable prioritizing patient care issues?* It would be appropriate to state "yes" and follow it with an example, such as, "I remember once, I had a patient with chest pain

and another patient who was bleeding. They both arrived at the same time. This is how I handled the situation ..." and give details.

- *Have you ever left a position because it was too "stressful"?* Be honest. If you have, admit it and explain why it was stressful. It would not be fair to you or to an employer to hire you if this was not the best job for you. Some offices and clinics are more stressful then others. A possible response would be: "I left the Northeast clinic because it was too stressful. I did not like caring for really young, sick children. I feel better taking caring of an older patient population."
- *How long do you think you will need for orientation?* If the office or clinic is in a staff crunch situation, you may be expected to work solo after a minimal orientation process. Again, be honest with your response. "I think that my skills are very strong and with a solid preceptor, I will be able to function independently within a few weeks."

Questions That Cannot Be Asked

Many questions legally cannot be asked during a job interview. State and federal laws regulate workplace discrimination. The United States Equal Employment Opportunity Commission (EEOC) enforces many of these laws. The three primary laws are Title VII, Americans with Disabilities Act (ADA), and the Age Discrimination in Employment Act (ADEA). It is illegal to ask any questions that could lead to discrimination based on a person's

- Race
- Color
- National origin
- Religion or religious beliefs
- Sex
- Age
- Disability
- Marital status
- Political affiliation
- Sexual orientation
- Pregnancy

There is an exception to this rule: A prospective employer may ask you any question if it is a bona fide occupational qualification. For example, it is illegal to ask some about religious beliefs, but you may be questioned about your religious beliefs towards abortion if you are applying to work in a clinic that performs abortions. If the job that you are applying for requires that you rotate shifts and holidays, a legal question would be, "As you know, this job requires that you work every Saturday morning. Will your family be ok if you work Saturdays?" The question does not directly ask if you are married, but the implication is obvious. Simply answer, "Yes, I will be able to work on Saturday mornings," and avoid the issue.

If you are asked an illegal question, you have two options. You can politely state, "I prefer not to answer that question." However, the reality is that you may not get the job, then you must decide if you want to pursue it through your local EEOC office. Your second option is to answer the question with a concise and direct answer. Whatever you do or say, maintain your professionalism. Be tactful.

Questions That You Should Ask

The interview should be a give-and-take situation. Just as the interviewer needs to determine whether you are suitable for the job, you need to know if this job will meet your needs.

Box 9-2   Questions That You Should Ask!

Here are some questions that you should ask during a job interview:
- Does this clinic have any other locations? Will I have to travel to them? If so, how often?
- Is your workforce stable? Do you anticipate any future layoffs?
- How soon will you want someone in place for this position?
- How long has this position been open?
- What is the salary range for this position? What are the shift differentials? Is there a pay increase with performance evaluations? What are the benefits? Will I be eligible for your health insurance plan?
- What are the hours for this position? Will they be consistent? What arrangements are made for holidays? What about weekends? Do we rotate weekends and holiday coverage? How does the rotation work? Is there an on-call schedule?
- Will I have to carry a beeper or pager? How often do I need to carry it?
- What is the staffing ratio? What other types of health care professionals will I be working with?
- How long will my orientation be?
- Do I need a physical examination before I start? Do you need proof of my immunizations?
- Will I be in charge of anyone? Will I work with licensed or unlicensed professionals? Who will be my supervisor?
- Is there an opportunity for overtime? Is overtime mandatory?
- How many applicants are being considered for this job?
- May I telephone you in 3-4 days to inquire about the position?
- Do you offer educational opportunities? Will you cover the expenses for me to attend educational seminars?
- When will I hear from you? When do you expect to make a decision?

Take a few moments to think about what questions you want to ask and then write the questions on a piece of paper *before* arriving for the interview (Box 9-2). Do not use a piece of notebook paper with ruffled edges. The paper should be neat and clean.

Generally, at the end of the interview, you will be asked, "Do you have any questions about this position or this office?" Then state, "Yes, I have written down a few questions." Ask your questions in a friendly and positive manner. Asking prewritten questions demonstrates professionalism and good organizational skills. Be conscious of your interviewer's time constraints. Watch for nonverbal cues that indicate the meeting is over.

Practical Tips for Surviving a Job Interview

There are many things you can do to make the interview a success. Here are 10 rules that you must follow to have a successful interview:
1. Be on time.
2. Be prepared.
3. Demonstrate confidence and maturity.
4. Pay attention to your posture. Sit straight. Walk with confidence. Do not shuffle.
5. Smile appropriately and always maintain eye contact.
6. Always provide a strong, solid handshake.
7. Learn as much about the job and facility as you can before the interview.
8. Keep the communication professional.

  9. Maintain a conversational tone.
10. Pay attention to detail.

Interviewing for a job is a skill that must be practiced over and over again. No one is perfect at interviewing the first time. You will be nervous. Mild nervousness and stress are actually beneficial, since they make you more alert and focused. However, when stress and anxiety hinder your ability to communicate effectively and professionally, that can cause you to lose employment opportunities. Most of the stress and anxiety you feel can be controlled through adequate preparation. Preparation should start weeks before the actual interview. Table 9-1 provides you with a pre-interview checklist that will help you prepare for interviewing.

Table **9-1   PRE-INTERVIEW CHECKLIST**

Here is a checklist to help you prepare for your interview. In the right hand column you will find a list of some items to do. Space has been provided for you to add your personal needs (such as arranging for babysitting, work, school).

At least 2 weeks before the interview, ask yourself these questions:	Do I have at least three solid references? Do I have the correct spelling of their names and titles? Do I know the correct addresses and telephone numbers of my references? Do I have enough copies of my resume, transcripts, awards, certifications, and diplomas?
At least 3 days before the interview, ask yourself these questions:	What outfit will I wear? (Be sure it is neatly ironed.) What shoes will I wear? Do I need new nylons? Do I have a clean, neat portfolio or brief case to bring with me? Do I know enough information about this hospital, clinic, or office?
The night before the interview:	Do I know how to get to the office? What time should I plan on leaving? (Plan plenty of time for parking and traffic.) Is my portfolio bag prepared? Plan to get plenty of rest. Did I review commonly asked questions? Am I comfortable with my responses? Do I have my list of questions typed or written out?
The day of the interview:	Avoid excessive caffeine ingestion. Avoid smoking (the smell will linger on your breath and clothes). Keep perfume to a minimum. Keep jewelry to a minimum. Fingernails should be short. Avoid brightly colored nail polish. Dress professionally.
Just before the interview:	Comb your hair in the bathroom, adjust your make-up. Sit quietly. Do not appear restless in your chair. Watch your nonverbal language. Avoid fidgeting. Complete an application as directed. Use a pen. Print neatly.

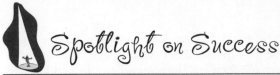

Spotlight on Success

Making your first impression requires appropriate clothing. It is not necessary to purchase an expensive business suit. For women, a nice skirt with a buttoned shirt and a blazer is appropriate. Closed-toe shoes with moderate heels are recommended. Keep make-up and jewelry to a minimum. Man should wear dress trousers, with a buttoned shirt and tie. If you are applying for a managerial position, a suit should be worn. Avoid using strong perfumes or cologne. A sharp, clean appearance puts you in the spotlight for future success.

Keep in mind as you go through the interview process that the employer must be certain that you are the right person for the position. Hiring the wrong person for a position is time consuming and costly and can be detrimental to patient care. Employers need to ask themselves a few questions before they decide to hire you:
- Are you a team player?
- Are you qualified? How long will your orientation need to be?
- Will your personality fit in with the other staff members?
- Are you dependable?
- If you have limited experience, are you worth the risk?
- Will you be happy working here? How long will you potentially stay? Will you be here in 6 months, a year, 5 years?

Be aware of these questions as you proceed through the interview process (see Spotlight on Success box; Fig. 9-4).

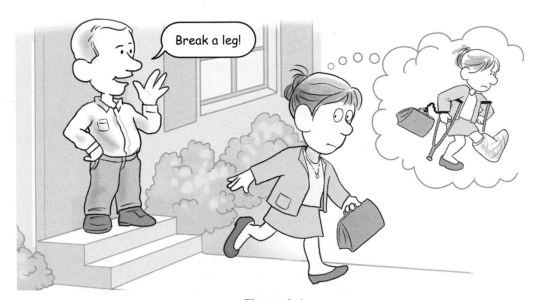

Figure 9-4

COMMUNICATION TOOL NUMBER FOUR: THE THANK-YOU LETTER

Now that the interview is over, you need to write a thank-you letter. A thank-you letter serves many purposes. First and foremost, it keeps your name and resume in the mind of the prospective employer. Quite often there are more applicants for a position than there are openings. You want your name to be on the top of the list.

Practical Tips for Writing a Thank-You Letter

The steps to writing a thank-you letter are similar to those of a cover letter. Take a few minutes to compose your thoughts, type the letter, and edit it. Be sure that your demographic information is the same as it was on your resume.

Timeliness

A thank-you letter should be sent promptly, within 1 to 2 business days. The prompt timing of a thank-you letter shows your prospective employer that you are an independent thinker and able to follow through on tasks. It also demonstrates courtesy, good organizational skills, and professionalism.

Body of the Letter

The first paragraph should consist of two or three sentences. It should start with a statement thanking the interviewer. Following that statement, indicate the position for which you are being considered. A brief sentence that you are excited about the position and are looking forward to joining the team should be third.

In the second paragraph, reemphasize your strengths and what you can bring to the position. Follow up or clarify any important issues. If you promised to send a document, this is a good place to refer to the enclosure. For example, "As promised, I am sending you a copy of my certification in cardiopulmonary resuscitation."

Two or three brief sentences are appropriate for your third paragraph. The intent of this paragraph is to indicate interest and to anticipate hearing about the position. State that you can be contacted for additional information if needed.

Use an appropriate closure term, such as "Sincerely," or "Regards," leave at least three spaces and then type your name. If you are including an enclosure, type "enc" underneath your typed name. If the enclosure is more than one page, put the number of pages being included in parenthesis. For example: enc (3). It is acceptable to write "enc" when sending just one page. Print the letter, sign it, place the letter and enclosures into a typed envelope and mail it (Fig. 9-5).

There are four communication tools you can use to get the job you desire. They are the resume, cover letter, interview, and thank-you letters. Learn to use each of these tools to their highest potential. Paying attention to the small details will increase your chance of acquiring your dream job.

Now that you have these tools, you can search for a job. Enlist the help of friends, peers, teachers, and school placement counselors. Your externship or clinical rotations are also good starting places.

Kathie Rubenstein

198 West Ice Cove

Willimington, Minnesota 559933

777-555-9999

E-mail: krubenstein@something.net

February 2, 2005

Shrel Abrahams

Clinical Supervisor

Minnesota Main Street Clinic

24 Sled Hill Road

Willimington, Minnesota 559933

Thank you for taking the time to meet with me yesterday. I am very interested in the medical assistant position that your clinic has open. I think the position sounds exciting and challenging.

My clinical skills are very strong and would be an asset to your clinic. In particular, my phlebotomy skills are very solid. I am comfortable drawing blood on all age groups. In addition, I can speak Spanish, which would also be an asset to your clinic population.

If you need any additional information, please feel free to contact me. I am looking forward to hearing from you about this position.

Sincerely,

Kathie Rubenstein

Figure 9-5
Thank-you letter.

Taking the Chapter to Work

Now, let's meet Aida and see how she has applied this chapter information in the workplace.

Today is Aida's last day as an extern and she decides to bring a small box of chocolates into the office. In addition, she has written a thank-you note to her preceptor and to the office manager. The thank-you note is sincere and personalized. She states in the note "Thank you for taking the time to improve my phlebotomy skills. I look forward to using these skills in the workforce. Enclosed is my phone number. Please keep me in mind if you have any job openings." Aida knows that at the present time the office does not have any job openings, but she wants to utilize every networking opportunity. Three months later Aida gets a surprise phone call from her externship site. An employee has just resigned and a job opening now exists. Aida quickly returns the call and accepts the job. Most health care jobs are never advertised. People are hired through networking. Start creating a strong network of friends.

B e y o n d the Classroom Exercises

Your Assignment Board

The following exercises will help you use your new knowledge. Place a check mark beside the assignments that your instructor has given you. When you have completed the assignment, place a check mark in the completed column.

		Assigned	*Completed*
Checking Your Comprehension	(Textbook)	☐	☐
Expanding Critical Thinking	(Textbook)	☐	☐
Communication Surfer Exercises	(Textbook and Internet)	☐	☐
Communication Branch #13	(CD-ROM)	☐	☐

Checking Your Comprehension

Write a brief answer to each of the following assignments.
1. Describe the five components of a resume.
2. List 10 action words that can be used in a resume.
3. What items should be included in the demographics section of a resume?
4. What is the purpose of a cover letter?
5. What is the purpose of thank-you letter? What is the recommended time frame for writing a thank-you letter?
6. Write five commonly asked interview questions and provide a good statement for each question.
7. List 10 topics that cannot legally be asked during a job interview.

Expanding Critical Thinking

1. What is a headhunter? What would you do if a headhunter called you? Would you refer a friend to a headhunter? Why or why not?
2. List 10 things you can do to remain calm during a job interview.
3. Write a cover and a thank-you letter. Then exchange yours with a friend. Did you find mistakes (grammar, punctuation, spelling)? When you get your letter back, correct your mistakes.
4. Write six good objectives for your resume.
5. Create a functional and a chronological resume for yourself.
6. Create a list of 15 possible questions that you may be asked in an interview. Write a good response for each question.
7. Describe your personality. Ask five friends to describe your personality. Compare the results. What characteristics are you happy with and which ones would you change? How can you improve yourself?

 ## Communication Surfer Exercises

1. Locate five resume help centers on the Internet. Create a list of at least 15 tips for creating a resume. Based on this information, which resume format is best for you? Why?
2. Locate three employment opportunities on the Internet. What words did you use on the search engine? What words helped you to narrow the search? Do you think the Internet is viable source to find a position? Why or why not? Create a sample cover letter for one of the positions.

Glossary

abbreviation   a shortened version of a complete word or phrase

acronym   a word formed by the initial letters of a series of words; e.g., ASAP ("as soon as possible")

adhere, adherence   to stick by, as in glue; to carry out a plan or scheme as directed

affective   concerned with feelings, emotions, or a mental state

algorithm   a step-by-step procedure for solving a problem or making a decision using a logical progression or protocol

amulet   an object, usually a necklace, worn as a charm against evil

anacusis   usually a total loss of hearing, but may indicate less severe hearing deficits

anticipatory grief   to foresee a traumatic event or occurrence and begin the process of coping

appease, appeased   to calm, satisfy, or relieve a situation by giving in to another

assess, assessment   to determine the significance or extent of a situation

assimilate, assimilation   to absorb into a whole, as in absorbing knowledge, or absorbing a socially distinct group into a dominant culture; the act or process of absorbing and retaining, as in information or other concepts

autonomy, autonomous   independent, self-governing

bariatric   a branch of medicine concerned with preventing, controlling, or treating obesity

belligerent, belligerence   hostile, aggressive, eager to fight

bereave, bereavement   to deprive or be deprived of something of value, usually by death

bias   a preference that inhibits impartial judgment

case conference   cohesive group of interdisciplinary professionals coming together to coordinate patient treatment

catatonic   usually a state of extreme immobility and muscle rigidity

chief compliant   a statement made by a patient describing the most significant or serious reason for concern

chronological resume   a method of listing progressive work experiences

clarify, clarifying, clarification   to make something easier to understand

cognition, cognitive   the process of knowing, including awareness, perception, reasoning, and judgment

cohesive, cohesion   the act or process of holding things together; a mutual attraction or joining of different entities

colloquialisms   informal speech, usually relying on regionally accepted terms and pronunciations

competency   verification of specific skill, knowledge, and/or ability for a given task

complement   something that completes or makes a thing whole; either of two parts that complete each other

compliant, compliance, complying   to yield to the command, requests, or wishes of another

consent form   form used to document patient permission before a procedure

consultation   to obtain advice or another opinion from a specialist regarding any aspect of patient care

cope, coping   contending or striving on more or less even terms or with success; to contend with difficulties and to overcome them

cover letter   a formal document that introduces a resume to a prospective employer

credible   capable of being believed

culture, cultural   a total collection of social behavior patterns, beliefs, and other community work and thought, characteristic of a certain population

delegating   process of assigning a project or task to someone

demographic   refers to personal identification information: name, address, telephone number

deny, denial   to reject or refuse to accept

discriminate, discrimination   to make a clear distinction or to differentiate, usually with negative perceptions

document, documentation   supplying written evidence or information for future reference

Do Not Resuscitate (DNR)   an order issued, usually at the request of the patient, not to use heroic, life-saving measures in the event of cardiac arrest

dynamics   the psychological background and inner workings of interpersonal relationships

emergent   a condition or situation that needs immediate attention; the failure to act quickly will result in a serious or untoward patient event

empathy   to identify with or understand the situation, feelings, or motives of another

endogenous   having its origins or originating within the body

escalate   increase, intensify

estrange, estrangement   to make hostile or unsympathetic; to terminate a relationship with negative feelings

ethnic, ethnicity   pertaining to a group joined by religion, race, nationality, or culture; the state of belonging to such a group

etiquette   the standard behavior that is acceptable in a given social, professional, or official setting

euphemism   substitution of an inoffensive term for one considered offensive

euphoria   a feeling of well-being or joy, usually exaggerated and not based on reality

eustress   good or positive stress with beneficial emotional and physical results

euthanasia   literally, "good death," implying that death is natural and easy and does not involve technological intervention; may be used to imply that death has been encouraged by medical means

evaluate, evaluation   to examine carefully to determine the condition of a thing or situation

exacerbate   to make worse or to increase in severity

exchange   in this instance, substituting an equal amount of one food for another of equal caloric value

exercise   in this instance, performed musculoskeletal activity to maintain fitness

exogenous   having its origins or origination outside of the body

feedback   the return of information solicited during an exchange; usually used to verify that information was received

flow sheet   form used to document routine and repetitive actions

functional resume   a method of listing skills or accomplishments in categories

gate, gating   to consciously block the reception of sensory stimuli, such as hearing or pain

graphic sheet   form used to document clinical items that can be plotted on a graph to show patient progress or deterioration

grief   deep mental anguish over a loss

holistic   considering the whole of a person, rather than treating one single aspect of the total person

idiom   an expression specific to a certain population that cannot be translated literally

impedance   a form of electrical resistance; in this instance, an interruption of sound transmission to the hearing centers of the brain

implement, implementation   a means of achieving a goal

imprudent   not wise or well considered

incident report   form used to communicate unusual events to supervisors, physicians, and risk management personnel

incongruent, incongruence   incompatible, not in agreement, inconsistent

inflection   alteration in pitch or tone of voice

interdependent   mutually dependent; a need for all parties to interact and depend on the others in the group

interdisciplinary   combination of two or more specialties working together to meet a specific goal

interview   a discussion or exchange to gather information, usually between two persons

intimidate, intimidating   to threaten, to discourage, or to inhibit

invincible, invincibility   incapable of being defeated

jargon   specialized or technical language of a trade or profession

kinesics   the study of body positions and movement in relation to communication

learning goal   the purpose toward which the gaining of specific knowledge or skill is directed

learning objective   an observable or discernible outcome as the result of acquired knowledge or information

maintain, maintenance   the act of preserving or keeping in an existing condition

maladaptive   failure to adjust or make necessary changes as a response to stress

manic   related to mania; and intense, possibly violent enthusiasm, interest, or desire

matriarch, matriarchal   a strong female figure; a society dominated by a strong female figure

message   a communication transmitted by spoken or written word or other means from one to another

military time   a 24-hour-clock system that allows each hour to be listed individually

mourn, mourning   the actions or expressions of one who is grieving

multitask   a term used by medical professionals who are required to do more than one thing at a time, in various situations, and do them safely

negative stress   stimuli that cause mental, physical, or emotional distress

noncompliant, noncompliance   failure or refusal by a patient to cooperate or follow medical instructions or advice

nonlanguage   communication methods other than spoken words, such as hums, sighs, chuckles, etc.

non-urgent   a condition or situation that needs to be addressed but it is not time dependent—the patient's outcome will not be worse if the condition is not resolved promptly

objective   a statement of goals or intentions

organic   in this instance, free of additives or synthetic chemicals

orient, orientation   adjusting or adapting to a new environment, situation, or set of ideas; introduction to a new situation

palliative   offering comfort, as in pain relief, but not bringing about a cure

paralanguage   vocal expression involving rate of speech, tone, pitch, etc.

paraphrase, paraphrasing   restating in other words or form than originally transmitted, usually to make a meaning clear

patient education   sharing information to allow a patient to understand health care as it relates to his situation

patriarch, patriarchal   a strong male figure; a society dominated by a strong male figure

peer   coworker

perpetuate, perpetuated   to cause to continue indefinitely

PIE   acronym used for documentation: *p*roblem, *i*mplementation, *e*valuation

plan, planning   to put together a program with a specific aim or purpose

positive stress   stimuli that result in beneficial physical, emotional, or mental changes

preparatory   introductory; to make ready

presbycusis   hearing deficits associated with the elderly

problem-oriented medical record (POMR)   charting system that divides charts into four sections: database, problem list, care plans, and progress notes

progress note   lined pages in a medical record that are used to document the patient's status

proxemics   the study of personal spatial distances and their effect on interpersonal behavior

prudent   careful in regard to one's own interests or conduct

psychomotor   movement associated with mental processes, as in planning and organizing musculoskeletal movements

quality improvement   process of identifying a problem, educating staff about the problem, and then reevaluating to see if the problem has improved or resolved

range of motion   the full degree of movement of a joint

rapport   a relationship, usually of mutual trust and regard

referral   a formal contract between two or more health care team members to provide services to a patient

reflect, reflecting   repeating back to the communicator the message that has been received, usually to ensure that the meaning is clear

regimen   a regulated program to promote health or other beneficial effect

regulatory agency   organization (private, federal, or state) that monitors health care settings for compliance with laws and standards—they can impose fines and/or close settings that do not adhere to the regulations.

reimbursement   payment made by an insurance company to a health care setting for medical services

reprisal   to pay back for a real or imagined injury

respite   a short interval of rest or relief

resume   a factual document that outlines professional and academic experiences

sedentary   accustomed to sitting or taking little exercise

sequence, sequential   one thing following another in an arrangement or order; forming a related series

SOAP, SOAPIE, SOAPIER   acronym used for documentation: *s*ubjective, *o*bjective, *a*ssessment, *p*lan, *i*mplementation, *e*valuation, *r*evision

source-oriented medical record (SOMR)   charting system that organizes the medical record into specialties

spatial   pertaining to a space and its relationship with things found in it

standard   a specific regulation or statement that depicts the minimum level of expected care

STAT   requiring an immediate response

stereotype, stereotyping   an oversimplification or broad grouping of persons or populations to fit a preconceived belief or opinion

subjective   existing in the mind; perceived only by the individual

summarize, summarizing   to restate in a briefer form

sympathy   a feeling or expression of pity or sorrow for the distress of another

template   an outline that allows the user to enter important information and create a document following an established format

thanatology   the study of dying and death and end-of-life issues

therapeutic   healing or curative

triage   process of sorting patients into categories based on level of illness

urgent   a condition or situation that needs quick and prompt attention—the failure to act within a reasonable timeframe could result in a deterioration of the patient's condition

validate, validating, validation   to verify that something is true

BIBLIOGRAPHY

Definitions for this glossary are adapted from the following sources:

The American Heritage Dictionary (3rd ed). (1992). Boston: Houghton-Mifflin.

Mosby's Medical, Nursing, and Allied Health Dictionary (6th ed). (2002). St. Louis, MO: Harcourt Health Sciences.

Appendix

COMMON ENGLISH-TO-SPANISH MEDICAL PHRASES

It is important to be able to communicate with all patients, regardless of their language. Learn a few phrases from languages that are commonly spoken in your geographic location. Consider taking a language course, preferably one designed for medical professionals.

This appendix contains common medical phrases translated from English into Spanish. For more information about communicating with Spanish-speaking patients, consult *Say It in Spanish: A Guide for Health Care Professionals* by Esperanza Villanueva Joyce and Maria Elena Villanueva, 3rd edition, (2004), Saunders.

GENERAL

Hi!	**¡Hola!** *(Oh-lah)*
Good morning.	**Buenos días.** *(Boo-eh-nohs dee-ahs)*
Good afternoon.	**Buenas tardes.** *(Boo-eh-nahs tahr-dehs)*
Good evening.	**Buenas noches.** *(Boo-eh-nahs noh-chehs)*
Good night.	**Buenas noches.** *(Boo-eh-nahs noh-chehs)*

Do you speak English?	¿Habla inglés? *(Ah-blah enn-glehs)*
No, I do not speak English.	No, no hablo inglés. *(Noh, noh ah-bloh een-glehs)*
Do you speak Spanish?	¿Habla español? *(Ah-blah ehs-pah-nyohl)*
Yes, I speak Spanish.	Sí, hablo español. *(See, ah-bloh ehs-pah-nyohl)*
No, I do not speak Spanish.	No, no hablo español. *(Noh, noh ah-bloh ehs-pah-nyohl)*
Yes, a little.	Sí, un poco. *(See, oon poh-koh)*
No, I don't understand.	No, no comprendo/no entiendo. *(Noh, noh kohm-prehn-doh/no ehn-tee-ehn-doh)*
Speak slowly, please.	Hable despacio, por favor. *(Ah-bleh dehs-pah-see-oh, pohr fah-bohr)*
What is your name?	¿Cómo se llama? *(Koh-moh seh yah-mah)*
What is your last name?	¿Cuál es su apellido? *(Koo-ahl ehs soo ah-peh-yee-doh)*
Answer "yes" or "no."	Conteste "sí" o "no". *(Kohn-tehs-teh "see" oh "noh")*
Do you have medical problems?	¿Tiene problemas médicos? *(Tee-eh-neh prohbleh-mahs meh-dee-kohs)*
Do you have pain?	¿Tiene dolor? *(Tee-eh-neh doh-lohr)*
I have pain.	Tengo dolor. *(Tehn-goh doh-lohr)*
The pain is on the side.	El dolor está en el lado/e costado. *(Ehl doh-lohr ehs-tah ehn ehl lah-doh/ eh kohs-tah-doh)*
The pain is localized, sharp.	El dolor está fijo, agudo. *(Ehl doh-lohr ehs tah fee-hoh, ah-goo-doh)*
The pain is worse.	El dolor es peor. *(Ehl doh-lohr ehs peh-ohr)*
I have nausea and fever.	Tengo náusea y fiebre. *(Tehn-goh nah-oo-seh-ah ee fee-eh-breh)*
Do you have high blood pressure?	¿Tiene presión alta? *(Tee-eh-neh preh-see-ohn ahl-tah)*
Do you have cardiac problems?	¿Tiene problemas cardíacos? *(Tee-eh-neh proh-bleh-mahs kahr-dee-ah-kohs)*
Do you feel weak?	¿Se siente débil? *(Seh see-ehn-teh deh-beel)*
Do you have chest pain?	¿Tiene dolor en el pecho? *(Tee-eh-neh doh-lohr ehn ehl peh-choh)*

Do you have a pace maker?	**¿Tiene marcapasos?** *(Tee-eh-neh mahr-kah-pah-sohs)*
Do you have allergies?	**¿Tiene alergias?** *(Tee-eh-neh ah-lehr-hee-ahs)*
Are you allergic to drugs?	**¿Es alérgico a drogas?** *(Ehs ah-lehr-hee-koh ah droh-gahs)*
Are you bleeding?	**¿Está sangrando?** *(Ehs-tah sahn-grahn-doh)*
Are you nauseated?	**¿Tiene náuseas?** *(Tee-eh-neh nah-oo-seh-ahs)*
Does the vomit have blood?	**¿Tiene sangre el vómito?** *(Tee-eh-neh sahn-greh ehl boh-mee-toh)*
Are you constipated?	**¿Está estreñido?** *(Ehs-tah ehs-treh-nyee-doh)*
Are you pregnant?	**¿Está embarazada?** *(Ehs-tah ehm-bah-rah-sah-dah)*
Have you had headaches?	**¿Ha tenido dolor de cabeza?** *(Ah teh-nee-doh doh-lohr deh kah-beh-sah)*
Have you passed out?	**¿Se ha desmayado?** *(Seh ah dehs-mah-yah-doh)*
Do you have dizzy spells?	**¿Tiene mareos?** *(Tee-eh-neh mah-reh-ohs)*
Swelling of the ankles?	**¿Hinchazón en los tobillos?** *(Eeh-chah-sohn ehn lohs toh-bee-yohs)*
Are you diabetic?	**¿Es diabético(a)** *(Ehs dee-ah-beh-tee-koh[ah])*
Do you drink alcohol?	**¿Toma bebidas alcohólicas?** *(Toh-mah beh-bee-dahs ahl-koh-lee-kahs)*
Does it hurt to breathe?	**¿Le duele al respirar?** *(Leh doo-eh-leh ahl rehs-pee-rahr)*
Does it hurt to cough?	**¿Le duele al toser?** *(Leh doo-eh-leh ahl toh-sehr)*
Does it hurts when I press?	**¿Duele cuando presiono?** *(Doo-eh-leh koo-ahn-doh preh-see-oh-noh)*
Has this happened before?	**¿Pasó esto antes?** *(Pah-soh ehs-toh ahn-tehs)*
Have you ever had cancer?	**¿Ha tenido cáncer?** *(Atl teh-nee-doh kahn-sehr)*

Have you had any bleeding,
   swelling, or bruising?
	¿Ha tenido sangrados, hinchazon moretones?
	*(Ah teh-nee-doh sahn-grah-dohs, een-chah-sohn,
	   oh moh-reh-toh-nehs)*

Have you had surgeries?	**¿Ha tenido operaciones?** *(Ah teh-nee-doh oh-peh-rah-see-ohn-ehs)*
Have you seen blood in the urine?	**¿Ha visto sangre en la orina?** *(Ah bees-toh sahn-greh ehn lah oh-ree-nah)*

What?	**¿Qué?/¿Qué tal?** *(Keh/keh tahl)*
When?	**¿Cuándo?** *(Koo-ahn-doh)*
Where?	**¿Dónde?** *(Dohn-deh)*
Why?	**¿Por qué?** *(Pohr keh)*
Who?	**¿Quién?** *(Kee-ehn)*
How many?	**¿Cuántos?** *(Koo-ahn-tohs)*
How much?	**¿Cuánto?** *(Koo-ahn-toh)*
Always!	**¡Siempre!** *(See-ehm-preh)*
Never!	**¡Nunca!** *(Noon-kah)*
Are you cold?	**¿Tiene frío?** *(Tee-eh-neh free-oh)*
Are you hot?	**¿Tiene calor?** *(Tee-eh-neh kah-lohr)*
Do you understand?	**¿Comprende/Entiende?** *(Kohm-prehn-deh/Ehn-tee-ehn-deh)*
Any questions?	**¿Alguna pregunta?** *(Ahl-goo-nah preh-goon-tah)*
I need to take your temperature and blood pressure.	**Necesito tomarle la temperatura y la presión de la sangre.** *(Neh-seh-see-toh toh-mahr-leh lah tehm-peh-rah-too-rah ee lah preh-see-ohn deh lah sahn-greh)*
I also need a urine sample.	**También necesito una muestra de orina.** *(Tahm-bee-ehn neh-seh-see-toh oo-nah moo-ehs-trah deh oh-ree-nah)*
You can go back to work in one week.	**Puede regresar al trabajo en una semana.** *(Poo-eh-deh reh-greh-sahr ahl trah-bah-hoh ehn oo nah seh-mah-nah)*
Sign here, please.	**Firme aquí, por tavor.** *(Feer-meh ah-kee, pohr fah-bohr)*
Thank you!	**¡Gracias!** *(Grah-see-ahs)*

COLORS

yellow	**amarillo** *(ah-mah-ree-yoh)*
amber	**a´mbar** *(ahm-bahr)*

clear   **claro**
                               (klah-roh)
white   **blanco**
                               (blahn-koh)
albino   **albino**
                               (ahl-bee-noh)
brown   **café**
                               (kah-feh)
black   **negro**
                               (neh-groh)
blue   **azul**
                               (ah-sool)
red   **rojo**
                               (roh-hoh)
green   **verde**
                               (behr-deh)

NUMBERS

1	one	**uno** *(oo-noh)*
2	two	**dos** *(dohs)*
3	three	**tres** *(trehs)*
4	four	**cuatro** *(koo-ah-troh)*
5	five	**cinco** *(seen-koh)*
6	six	**seis** *(seh-ees)*
7	seven	**siete** *(see-eh-teh)*
8	eight	**ocho** *(oh-choh)*
9	nine	**nueve** *(noo-eh-beh)*
10	ten	**diez** *(dee-ehs)*
11	eleven	**once** *(ohn-seh)*
12	twelve	**doce** *(doh-seh)*
13	thirteen	**trece** *(treh-seh)*

14	fourteen	**catorce**
		(kah-tohr-seh)
15	fifteen	**quince**
		(keen-seh)
16	sixteen	**dieciséis**
		(dee-ehs-ee-seh-ees)
17	seventeen	**diecisiete**
		(dee-ehs-ee-see-eh-teh)
18	eighteen	**dieciocho**
		(dee-ehs-ee-oh-choh)
19	nineteen	**diecinueve**
		(dee-ehs-ee-noo-eh-beh)
20	twenty	**veinte**
		(beh-een-teh)

PHLEBOTOMY

The doctor ordered blood samples.	**El doctor/La doctora ordeno muestras de sangre.**
	(Seh-nyoh-rah Gahr-sah, ehl dohk-tohr/lah dohk-toh-rah ohr-deh-noh moo-ehs-trahs deh sahn-greh)
I am here to draw your blood.	**Estoy aquí para tomarile una muestra de sangre.**
	(Ehs-toh-ee ah-kee pah-rah toh-mahr-leh oo-nah moo-ehs-trah deh sahn-greh)
I am going to lift your sleeve.	**Voy a levantar la manga.**
	(Boh-ee ah leh-bahn-tahr lah mahn-gah)
Make a fist.	**Cierre la mano. Haga un puño.**
	(See-eh-reh lah mah-noh/Ah-gah oon poo-nyoh)
Open your hand.	**Abra la mano.**
	(Ah-brah lah mah-noh)
I want to take a sample from your finger.	**Quiero tomar una muestra del dedo.**
	(Kee-eh-roh toh-mahr oo-nah moo-ehs-trah dehl deh-doh)
I want to see the sugar level.	**Quiero ver el nivel de azúcar.**
	(Kee-eh-roh behr ehl nee-behl deh ah-soo-kahr)
This is done quickly.	**Esto se hace rápido.**
	(Ehs-toh seh ah-seh rah-pee-doh)
Have you had blood drawn before?	**¿Le han tomado muestras de sangre antes?**
	(Leh ahn toh-mah-doh moo-ehs-trahs deh sahn-greh ahn-tehs)
I need two tubes of blood:	**Necesito dos tubos de sangre:**
	(Neh-seh-see-toh dohs too-bohs deh sahn-greh)
One tube for a blood count.	**Un tubo para una biometría hemática.**
	(Oon too-boh pah-rah oo-nah bee-oh-meh-tree-ah eh-mah-tee kah)
Another for a serology test.	**Otro para una prueba serológica.**
	(Oh-troh pah-rah oo-nah proo-eh bah seh-roh-loh-hee-kah)

I need to use a tourniquet.
Necesito usar un torniquiete.
(Neh-seh-see-toh oo-sahr oon tohr-nee-keh-teh)

I am going to put a Band-Aid on you.
Voy a ponerle una cinta adhesiva/una curita/un bandaid.
(Boh-ee ah poh-nehr-leh oo-nah seen-tah ah-deh-see-bah/oo-nah koo-ree-tah/oon bahn-dah-eed)

Please, bend your arm for about five minutes.
Por favor, doble el brazo por cinco minutos.
(Pohr fah-bohr, doh-bleh ehl brah-soh pohr seen-koh mee-noo-tohs)

MEDICATION

Do you take any medicines?
¿Toma algunas medicinas?
(Toh-mah ahl-goo-nahs meh-dee-see-nahs)

What medicines do you take?
¿Qué medicinas toma?
(Keh meh-dee-see-nahs toh-mah)

For what reason?
¿Cuál es la razón?
(Koo-ahl ehs lah rah-sohn)

Are you taking your medicines?
¿Está tomando sus medicinas?
(Ehs-tah toh-mahn-doh soos meh-dee-see-nahs)

Are you allergic to drugs?
¿Es alérgico a drogas?
(Ehs ah-lehr-hee-koh ah droh-gahs)

Take the medicine with juice.
Tome la medicina con jugo.
(Toh-meh lah meh-dee-see-nah kohn hoo-goh)

Take it with a full glass of water.
Tómela con un vaso lleno de agua.
(Toh-meh-lah kohn oon bah-soh yeh-noh dehah-goo-ah)

Do not drink alcohol with this medicine.
No tome alcohol con esta medicina.
(No toh-meh ahl-kohl kohn ehs-tah meh-dee-see-nah)

It can cause drowsiness.
Le puede causar sueño.
(Leh poo-eh-deh kah-oo-sahr soo-eh-nyoh)

Do not drive!
¡No maneje/conduzca!
(Noh mah-neh-heh/kohn-doos-kah)

Take the medicine with food.
Tome la medicina con comida.
(Toh-meh lah meh-dee-see-nah kohn koh-mee-dah)

Avoid sunlight.
Evite asolearse/los rayos del sol.
(Eh-bee-teh ah-soh-leh-ahr-seh/lohs rah-yohs dehl sohl)

Follow the instructions carefully.
Siga las instrucciones con cuidado.
(See-gah lahs eens-trook-see-ohn-ehs kohn koo-ee-dah-doh)

This medicine is a pain killer.
Esta medicina quita/alivia el dolor.
(Ehs-tah meh-dee-see-nah kee-tah/ah-lee-bee-ah ehl doh-lohr)

Take on an empty stomach.
Tómela con el estómago vacío.
(Toh-meh-lah kohn ehl ehs-toh-mah-goh bah-see-oh)

Take one hour before eating.
Tómela una hora antes de comer.
(Toh-meh-lah oo-nah oh-rah ahn-tehs deh koh-mehr)

Three times a day.

Tres veces al día.
(Trehs beh-sehs ahl dee-ah)

Twice a day.

Dos veces al día.
(Dohs beh-sehs ahl dee-ah)

Daily.

Diariamente./Una por día./Cada día.
(Dee-ah-ree-ah-mehn-teh/Oo-nah pohr dee-ah/Kah-dah dee-ah)

Before/after meals.

Antes/después de las comidas.
(Ahn-tehs/dehs-poo-ehs deh lahs koh-mee-dahs)

At bedtime.

Al acostarse./A la hora de dormir.
(Ahl ah-kohs-tahr-seh/Ah lah oh-rah deh dohr-meer)

You can refill _____ times.

Puede surtir _____ veces.
(Poo-eh-deh soor-teer _____ beh-sehs)

Take all the medicine in the prescription.

Tome toda la medicina indicada en la receta.
(Toh-meh toh-dah lah meh-dee-see-nah een-dee-kah-dah ehn lah reh-seh-tah)

This prescription may not be refilled.

Esta receta no se puede surtir de nuevo.
(Ehs-tah reh-seh-tah noh seh poo-eh-deh soor-teer deh noo-eh-boh)

PEDIATRICS

Has the child been ill?

¿Ha estado enfermo el niño?
(Ah ehs-tah-doh ehn-fehr-moh ehl nee-nyoh)

Sleeping well?

¿Durmiendo bien?
(Door-mee-ehn-doh bee-ehn)

Breast feeding?

¿Tomando pecho?
(Toh-mahn-doh peh-choh)

Taking formula?

¿Tomando fórmula?
(Toh-mahn-doh fohr-moo-lah)

What formula does he take?

¿Qué fórmula toma?
(Keh fohr-moo-lah toh-mah)

How many ounces does he take?

¿Cuántas onzas toma?
(Koo-ahn-tahs ohn-sahs toh-mah)

How often do you feed the baby?

¿Qué tan a menudo alimenta al bebé?
(Keh tahn ah meh-noo-doh ah-lee-mehn-tah ahl beh-beh)

Does the baby sleep all night?

¿Duerme el bebé toda la noche?
(Doo-ehr-meh ehl beh-beh toh-dah lah noh-cheh)

How many times does he wake up?

¿Cuántas veces se despierta?
(Koo-ahn-tahs beh-sehs seh dehs-pee-ehr-tah)

Does he cry a lot?

¿Llora mucho?
(Yoh-rah moo-choh)

When was the last time he had a bowel movement?

¿Cuándo fué la última vez que evacuó/hizo del baño?
(Koo-ahn-doh foo-eh lah ool-tee-mah behs keh eh-bah-koo-oh/ee-soh dehl bah-nyoh)

Is he urinating well?

¿Orina bien?
(Oh-ree-nah bee-ehn)

Have you seen blood in
the urine?

¿Ha visto sangre en la orina?
(Ah bees-toh sahn-greh ehn lah oh-ree-nah)

How many diapers have you
changed since yesterday?

¿Cuántos pañales le ha cambiado desde ayer?
(Koo-ahn-tohs pah-nyah-lehs leh ah kahm-bee-ah-doh
dehs-deh ah-yehr)

Is he coughing?

¿Está tosiendo?
(Ehs-tah toh-see-ehn-doh)

Does he cough only at night?

¿Tose sólo de noche?
(Toh-seh soh-loh deh noh-cheh)

Do any of your children
have asthma?

¿Algunos de sus niños tienen asma?
(Ahl-goo-nohs deh soos nee-nyohs tee-eh-nehn ahs-mah)

Cold/flu?

¿Resfriado/gripa?
(Rehs-free-ah-doh/gree-pah)

Chickenpox?

¿Varicela?
(Bah-ree-seh-lah)

You can feed him/her
solid foods.

Puede darle alimentos sólidos.
(Poo-eh-deh dahr-leh ah-lee-mehn-tohs soh-lee-dohs)

From Joyce, E.V. and Villanueva, M.E. (2004). *Say It in Spanish: A Guide for Health Care Professionals*, 3rd ed.
St. Louis: Saunders.

Index

Note: Page numbers followed by f indicate figures; those followed by t indicate tables; those followed by b indicate boxed material.